101 Weight Loss Tips

for Preventing and Controlling Diabetes

Anne Daly, MS, RD, BC-ADM, CDE

Linda Delahanty, MS, RD, LD

Judith Wylie-Rosett , EdD, RD

American Diabetes Association.

*Cure • Care • Commitment*SM

Director, Book Publishing, John Fedor; *Book Acquisitions*, Sherrye Landrum; *Editor,* Sherrye Landrum; *Production Manager,* Peggy M. Rote; *Composition*, Circle Graphics, Inc.; *Cover Design*, Bremmer & Goris Communications; *Printer,* Transcontinental Printing

Printed in Canada
1 3 5 7 9 10 8 6 4 2

The suggestions and information contained in this publication are generally consistent with the *Clinical Practice Recommendations* and other policies of the American Diabetes Association, but they do not represent the policy or position of the Association or any of its boards or committees. Reasonable steps have been taken to ensure the accuracy of the information presented. However, the American Diabetes Association cannot ensure the safety or efficacy of any product or service described in this publication. Individuals are advised to consult a physician or other appropriate health care professional before undertaking any diet or exercise program or taking any medication referred to in this publication. Professionals must use and apply their own professional judgment, experience, and training and should not rely solely on the information contained in this publication before prescribing any diet, exercise, or medication. The American Diabetes Association—its officers, directors, employees, volunteers, and members—assumes no responsibility or liability for personal or other injury, loss, or damage that may result from the suggestions or information in this publication.

⊗ The paper in this publication meets the requirements of the ANSI Standard Z39.48-1992 (permanence of paper).

ADA titles may be purchased for business or promotional use or for special sales. For information, please write to Lee Romano Sequeira, Special Sales & Promotions, at the address below.

American Diabetes Association
1701 North Beauregard Street
Alexandria, Virginia 22311

Library of Congress Cataloging-in-Publication Data

Daly, Anne, 1951-
  101 weight loss tips for preventing and controlling diabetes / by Anne Daly, Linda Delahanty, Judith Wylie-Rosett.
    p. cm.
Includes index.
  ISBN 1-58040-132-5 (pbk. : alk. paper)
  1. Diabetes—Popular works. 2. Weight loss—Popular works. I. Title: One hundred one weight loss tips for preventing and controlling diabetes. II. Title: One hundred and one weight loss tips for preventing and controlling diabetes. III. Title: Weight loss tips for preventing and controlling diabetes. IV. Delahanty, Linda. V. Wylie-Rosett, Judy. VI. Title.
  RC600.4 .D355 2002
  616.4′620654—dc21

                                                                              2002018576

Contents

▼

INTRODUCTION

▼

Too often people are just told to "lose weight." Where do you begin? Is it worth the effort? Can you succeed? Yes, you can, and this book can help you do it. Any approach to losing weight needs to be simple and organized. We have found that it helps to expand your focus to four areas of your life: Weight, Activity, Variety, and Excess (WAVE). Yes, weight is the subject of this book, but the discussion must be about ways to increase activity and variety and to reduce excess in all areas. In other words, eat in moderation. Exercise in moderation. Feel stress in moderation. As for "why" you want to lose weight, it's more than looking and feeling better. Losing weight can prevent health problems such as high blood pressure and diabetes. If you already have diabetes, weight loss can help you control it.

The Weight section of this book addresses the basics of losing weight and maintaining it, concerns if you have diabetes or are trying to keep from getting it, and surgery and medications for weight loss. The Activity section has three chapters on the basics, exercise and diabetes complications, and community changes to make being physically active easier. The Variety section has two chapters to help you plan for success and eating out. The Excess section talks about what to do when your environment is out of control, emotions, and roadblocks to success.

The WAVE concept was developed by the Practice and Patient Materials Committee from a consortium of 21 medical schools with Nutrition Academic Award funding. It is a useful way for health providers to work with you to achieve a healthier lifestyle and manage your weight.

SECTION I
Weight

Chapter 1
THE BASICS

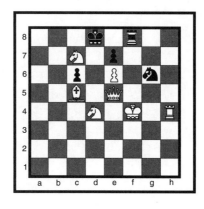

*W*hat are my health benefits if I lose weight?

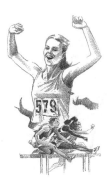

▼
TIP:

If you lose weight, you can reduce your risk of getting diabetes, heart disease, high blood pressure, gall bladder disease, and breast and colon cancer. If you already have any of these health problems, losing weight improves them. When you lose weight, you'll spend less time and money on doctor's visits and health problems.

People who lose even small amounts of weight—5–7% of their starting weight (usually 10–20 pounds) improve their health by reducing high blood pressure, high blood sugar, high cholesterol, sleep apnea, arthritis, and depression. And their self-esteem grows. Even without weight loss, you start getting health benefits just as soon as you take steps to improve your lifestyle with a meal plan and more physical activity. Just do it.

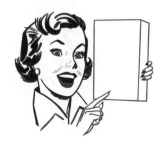

Which weight table should I use to find my healthy body weight?

TIP:

Since being overweight is associated with increased risk of death, the life insurance industry has been making the public aware of it. The 1959 and 1983 Metropolitan Life Insurance Company tables of ideal body weight are still among the most popular in use, but they are very strict. In 1990, the federal government issued an updated table of suggested weights for adults based on height and age—the BMI table, which lists reasonable body weights. There is no "ideal" body weight.

Body Mass Index (BMI) Values

BMI

Height	Good Weights								27					Increasing Risk								
	19	**20**	**21**	**22**	**23**	**24**	**25**	**26**	**27**	**28**	**29**	**30**	**31**	**32**	**33**	**34**	**35**	**36**	**37**	**38**	**39**	**40**
										Weight (in pounds)												
4'10"	91	96	100	105	110	115	119	124	129	134	138	143	148	153	158	162	167	172	177	181	186	191
4'11"	94	99	104	109	114	119	124	128	133	138	143	148	153	158	163	168	173	178	183	188	193	198
5'	97	102	107	112	118	123	128	133	138	143	148	153	158	163	168	174	179	184	189	194	199	204
5'1"	100	106	111	116	122	127	132	137	143	148	153	158	164	169	174	180	185	190	195	201	206	211
5'2"	104	109	115	120	126	131	136	142	147	153	158	164	169	175	180	186	191	196	202	207	213	218
5'3"	107	113	118	124	130	135	141	146	152	158	163	169	175	180	186	191	197	203	208	214	220	225
5'4"	110	116	122	128	134	140	145	151	157	163	169	174	180	186	192	197	204	209	215	221	227	232
5'5"	114	120	126	132	138	144	150	156	162	168	174	180	186	192	198	204	210	216	222	228	234	240
5'6"	118	124	130	136	142	148	155	161	167	173	179	186	192	198	204	210	216	223	229	235	241	247
5'7"	121	127	134	140	146	153	159	166	172	178	185	191	198	204	211	217	223	230	236	242	249	255
5'8"	125	131	138	144	151	158	164	171	177	184	190	197	203	210	216	223	230	236	243	249	256	262
5'9"	128	135	142	149	155	162	169	176	182	189	196	203	209	216	223	230	236	243	250	257	263	270
5'10"	132	139	146	153	160	167	174	181	188	195	202	209	216	222	229	236	243	250	257	264	271	278
5'11"	136	143	150	157	165	172	179	186	193	200	208	215	222	229	236	243	250	257	265	272	279	286
6'	140	147	154	162	169	177	184	191	199	206	213	221	228	235	242	250	258	265	272	279	287	294
6'1"	144	151	159	166	174	182	189	197	204	212	219	227	235	242	250	257	265	272	280	288	295	302
6'2"	148	155	163	171	179	186	194	202	210	218	225	233	241	249	256	264	272	280	287	295	303	311
6'3"	152	160	168	176	184	192	200	208	216	224	232	240	248	256	264	272	279	287	295	303	311	319
6'4"	156	164	172	180	189	197	205	213	221	230	238	246	254	263	271	279	287	295	304	312	320	328

BMI ≥27 are highlighted because health risk escalates rapidly above this level.

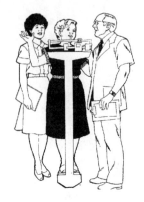

What is reasonable body weight?

▼

TIP:

Reasonable body weight is a term that appears in the *1994 Nutrition Recommendations for People with Diabetes*. This is defined as the weight that you and your health care team agree that you can probably achieve and maintain for the rest of your life. This weight turns out to be very different from ideal body weight, but it does reduce your health risks. For instance, a female who is 5'5" tall has an ideal body weight on the outdated table of 120 lbs. In real life however, if her current weight is 220, a reasonable body weight for her might be 160 lbs.

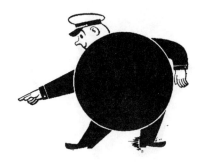

*H*ow do I know if I'm overweight or obese?

▼
TIP:

Overweight and obesity are related but do not mean the same thing. Overweight refers to an excess amount of body weight for your height that includes all tissues, such as fat, bone, muscle, and water. For example, a football player with a lot of muscle might weigh a lot but it isn't fat that makes him weigh so much. Obesity refers to an excess of body fat. You can measure obesity using the body mass index (BMI).

Category	Body Mass Index
Underweight	<18.5
Normal	18.5–24.9
Overweight	25.0–29.9
Obesity	30.0–34.9
Severe Obesity	35.0–39.9
Morbid Obesity	≥40.0

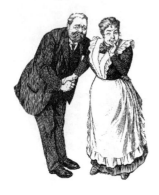

*H*ow do I calculate my BMI?

▼

TIP:

Body mass index or BMI is a way to measure overweight or obesity based on weight and height.

BMI = weight in kilograms / height in meters^2. To calculate your BMI, you need to know your height and your weight.
Your weight in pounds divided by 2.2 = your weight in kilograms.

For example, if you weigh 200 pounds, then you weigh 90.9 kilograms.

$$\frac{200}{2.2} = 90.9$$

Your height in inches $\times$ 2.54 = your height in centimeters. Divide your height in centimeters by 100 to get your height in meters.

If you are 68 inches tall, then you are 172.7 centimeters or 1.727 meters tall.

$$68 \times 2.54 = \frac{172.7}{100} = 1.727$$

$$\text{Your BMI would be } \frac{90.9}{1.727 \times 1.727} = 30.5$$

This BMI says that you meet the criteria for obesity, and you may have some serious health problems.

*H*ow does BMI relate to health risk?

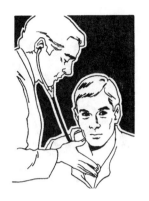

▼
TIP:

The health problems that come along with obesity are coronary heart disease, stroke, high blood pressure, sleep apnea, diabetes, gout, high cholesterol, arthritis, and gallstones. All overweight and obese adults (ages 18 years or older) with a BMI of 25 or higher are at risk for developing these health problems. Those with a BMI of 30 or higher have serious health risks, especially for heart disease. When you lose weight, you improve your health in many ways!

BMI	Health Risk Based on BMI	Risk if you have other health problems
<25	Minimal	Low
25–<27	Low	Moderate
27–<30	Moderate	High
30–<35	High	Very high
35–<40	Very high	Extremely high
≥40	Extremely high	Extremely high

Obese people may be limited in how agile they are, so they have a higher risk of having accidents. They may have difficulty getting pregnant and difficulties with pregnancy and delivery. You and your doctor should consider all of your health problems when choosing a weight loss program. NOTE: You are more likely to have health risks when your body fat is concentrated in your belly rather than in your hips. To check the location of your body fat use the waist-to-hip measurement (page 10).

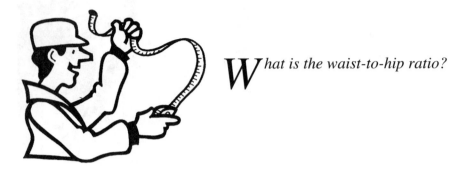

*W*hat is the waist-to-hip ratio?

▼
TIP:

The waist-to-hip ratio (WHR) is the comparison of your waist measurement to your hip measurement. It is a way to see whether your weight is primarily in your hips and buttocks (in what is known as a "pear" shape, common in females) or in the abdomen (making an "apple" shape, common in males). Measure your waist with a nonstretchable measuring tape at the smallest point (between the rib cage and navel), and measure your hips at the widest point (around the buttocks). A WHR of more than 1.0 in males and 0.8 in females suggests that you have increased health risks. As an example, a woman who weighs 300 lbs has a waist measuring 53 inches and hip measuring 60 inches.

$$\frac{53}{60} = .9$$

The waist/hip ratio is 0.9.

The risk is higher for women with a waist measurement of 35 inches or more and higher for men with a waist measurement 40 inches or more.

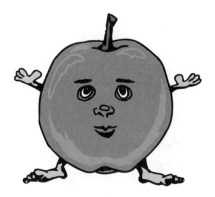

I *tend to have a belly. Is being*
shaped like an apple bad?

Yes, because where your body stores fat makes a difference in your health. People who have a larger waist are more likely to develop heart disease, high blood pressure, and diabetes. Health risks seem to come with having a waist measurement of greater than 35 inches in women and greater than 40 inches in men. Abdominal fat is worse than fat on your buttocks or thighs, because that extra fat surrounds important organs such as the liver and pancreas. When you have fat in this area of the body, your body can't use the insulin produced by your pancreas very well. This is called insulin resistance, and it causes high blood sugar levels. High blood sugar levels put your organs at higher risk.

If you lose weight, the amount of fat stored around your waist and important organs will decrease, and they will all work better.

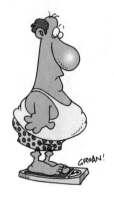

GROAN!

Everybody in my family is heavy. How can I ever expect to be thin?

▼

TIP:

You may not ever be thin, but you can certainly lose weight and get fit. It may help to think of your family's gift this way: you may have inherited genes that make you more energy efficient. People who survive a famine are likely to have a "thrifty gene" that allows them to get by on fewer calories. When the food supply is more plentiful, people who are more energy efficient gain weight.

The second thing you inherit from your family is your lifestyle. When the Pima Indians, who had low rates of obesity until 50 years ago, adopted the "Western" lifestyle, food was plentiful and they exercised less. They now have an epidemic of obesity and diabetes.

Families pass on habits that may lead to weight gain. Your parents played a strong role in the development of your food preferences, physical activity habits, and eating habits. But you can make new habits. And pass them on to your children, too.

Chapter 2
WEIGHT LOSS

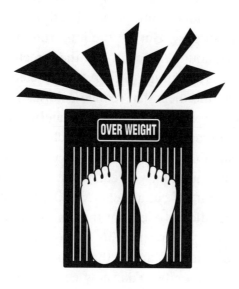

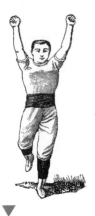

Is one method of losing weight better than the other?

TIP:

Yes, eating fewer calories than you burn is the key. There are a variety of weight loss therapies ranging from nutrition therapy (low-calorie diets and increasing physical activity) to behavior therapy, drugs, and surgery. But for the long run, it's burning the calories you eat that counts. Recently, at the direction of NIH, the U.S. Department of Agriculture (USDA) completed a study on popular diets and found the diets that reduce calories result in weight loss. If you don't exercise, eating approximately 1,400–1,500 calories a day is recommended, no matter which foods you eat.

It is also appears that the easiest way to control calories is by cutting back on how much fat you eat. Most people who succeed at weight loss and keep it off eat a diet with 20–30% of their calories from fat. This is significantly less fat than is in the average American diet, which is more than 36% calories from fat.

What you need to understand is that you don't follow a diet for 8 days, 8 weeks, or 8 months. Your new eating habits are the basis of your everyday food choices for the rest of your life. Healthy meal plans are high in vegetables, fruits, and other carbohydrates such as whole grains and low-fat dairy products. This is a moderate-fat, low-calorie way of eating that stops weight gain, leads to weight loss, and keeps it off. It is fast, convenient, and inexpensive. So— why are people still looking for a magic pill? This tastes better!

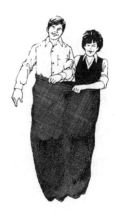

*W*hy do I need to be physically active?

To burn the calories you eat. We gain weight when we take in more food energy than we use up. Being physically active makes you healthier because all your systems—heart, lungs, circulation, and digestion—get exercise, too. But being active is particularly helpful to people who want to lose weight, because it burns calories. You get a 1-pound weight loss for every 3,500 calories burned. Exercise also helps you build muscle. Building muscle is good because it burns calories even when you are at rest. People with diabetes benefit from exercise, because it lowers blood glucose, too.

Exercise benefits are many and include:

- More energy
- Weight loss
- Improved mobility and range of motion
- A better attitude and self-esteem
- Better blood glucose control
- Reduced chance of heart attack or stroke
- Improved blood pressure
- Improved cholesterol levels

Please remember muscle weighs more than fat. While you are building muscle and losing fat, don't wail at the scale. Measure the inches you're losing on waist, thigh, and biceps to see your progress at weight loss.

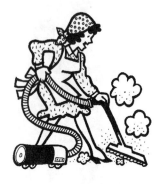

*H*ow can I burn more calories?

▼
TIP:

You may be surprised at how many of your daily activities burn calories. This table shows the calories burned by a 150-pound person doing 30 minutes of each activity. If you weigh more than 150, you will burn more calories.

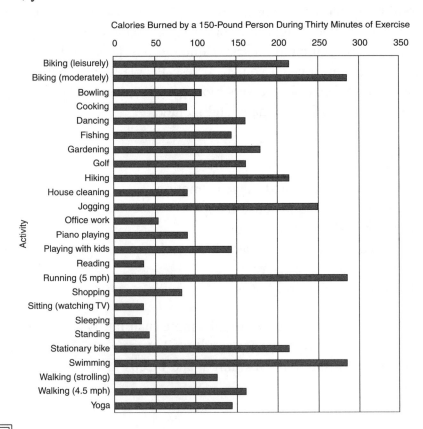

Calories Burned by a 150-Pound Person During Thirty Minutes of Exercise

*W*hat about the popular fad diets— do they work?

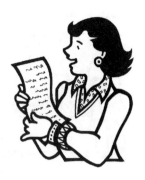

▼
TIP:

Not really. At the beginning, these diets may produce some weight loss, but you are losing water weight. The other reason they work at first is that these diets are, basically, low-calorie diets in disguise. When you follow them closely, these diets typically provide 1,000–1,600 calories daily. For most Americans, this is fewer calories than they usually eat. However, the problem is maintaining the weight loss. These diets are hard to stick with. You soon miss carbohydrate foods and wander back to old eating habits. Almost all the popular diets promote eating high protein and low carbohydrate. The authors claim that you can eat unlimited amounts of high protein and high-fat foods, but they severely limit fruits, vegetables, legumes, whole grain and milk products, breads, cereal, and crackers. Hey folks, those are the healthiest foods! There is a long list of serious health risks associated with these diets, such as poor nutrition, increased blood pressure, increased blood cholesterol, cancer, osteoporosis, gout, and kidney stones. For people with diabetes, these diets are particularly bad because eating lots of saturated fat puts you at risk for heart attack and stroke.

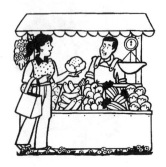

*W*hat can I do instead of the popular diets to lose weight successfully?

▼
TIP:

There are no quick fixes to losing weight. Simply put, you need to burn more calories than you take in. To help you do that, follow these guidelines:

- Eat a varied diet—include all food groups
- Include at least 5 servings of fruits and vegetables daily
- Limit sugary foods
- Eat smaller servings
- Limit fat, especially saturated (animal) fat and trans fats (in hydrogenated oils)
- Be physically active at least 30 minutes 3–5 days of the week

Seek help from a registered dietitian (RD), preferably one who is a certified diabetes educator (CDE), if you have diabetes, to develop a meal plan based on your likes and dislikes, daily schedule, and health concerns. This is a very important step in creating a healthier lifestyle.

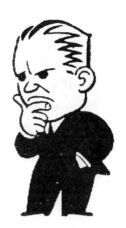

*W*hat should I consider when choosing
a weight management program?

▼
TIP:

*A*sk yourself these questions about the program:

- How often do I go and how long are the sessions?
- Is the program conveniently located and does the time fit my schedule?
- What are my short-term and my long-term goals?
- Do I have high health risks?
- Is my health checked at the beginning and monitored throughout the program?
- Is the staff trained and experienced in treating my medical condition(s)?
- What method(s) are used for weight loss? Are there expensive foods to buy?
- Does the program include instruction in healthful eating, increasing physical activity, and improving self-esteem?
- Once I lose the weight, what services are provided for long-term maintenance?
- Do they have records to show their success with both weight loss and maintenance?
- What medical standards does the staff follow to care for my health conditions?
- What type(s) of ongoing support do they provide me?
- Are there any possible health risks or side effects for me to be aware of?
- What are the costs, and are any covered by insurance?

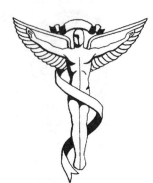

*W*hat is a "state-of-the-art" weight management program?

The best program is like the lifestyle-change one used to prevent diabetes in the Diabetes Prevention Program (DPP). Lifestyle-change patients had a daily goal for grams of total fat. If meeting that goal did not help them lose weight, they worked on eating 1,200–1,800 calories a day, with less than 25% of calories from fat. Patients were asked to do 30 minutes of moderate physical activity, such as brisk walking, at least 5 days a week. For support and education, they attended 16 individual sessions over 6 months and group sessions with 10–20 others. The lifestyle-change staff was a team of professionals, including RDs, exercise physiologists, and behaviorists. Participants kept daily records of calories and physical activity (minutes or calories burned). Most patients completed the 3-year study, reaching their lifestyle goals. The results were dramatic: 58% of those in the lifestyle-change group prevented diabetes, compared to 31% of those who just took medication. The state-of-the-art program gives you goals for daily fat grams, calorie range, physical activity, and record keeping, and provides you with professional support, in both individual and group sessions.

A re food records really necessary—
if so, why?

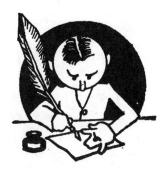

▼
TIP:

Y es. This is one of the best weight loss techniques. If you write
down what you eat and drink, you are more likely to succeed
at weight loss and weight maintenance. Food records give you the
history of what you've eaten, so that your weight loss—or weight
gain—is no mystery. Besides that, food records give you something
real to work with. You can identify problems, and you can begin to
problem-solve. Without records, you won't even know what the
problems are. Record keeping helps you monitor your progress and
skill level, and identify patterns in your weight management behavior. The feedback from your records strengthens your skills for
weight management. Write down foods within 15 minutes of eating.
Most successful record keepers total their numbers at the end of the
day or the first thing the next morning on a weekly summary sheet.
Keeping good records is a skill that takes lots of practice to develop.
There will be stops and starts, and most people do not enjoy keeping records, because they take work. But it is really worthwhile
work. You will benefit from it!

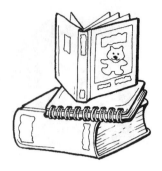

*W*hat do food records look like, and what do I do with them?

Y ou can keep your records in a spiral notebook or on cards or however you want to do it. Your records need columns or places to write the name of food, the serving size (ounces, cups, tablespoons), and the calories or fat grams or carbohydrate grams of servings or exchange groups, depending on which meal planning method you use. For weight management, you can track the number of servings of vegetables and fruits you eat per day—and aim for 5 or more (3 veggies, 2 fruits). At the end of a week, you can add up your weekly totals of calories, vegetable servings, fruit servings, etc. From those totals, you can figure your average daily calorie, carbohydrate, and fat intake. Make a column for anything else that has an impact on your food choices or eating behavior during the day. You should note the time you eat, where you are, whom you're with, and if anything is causing tension around you. You should note your daily exercise—even if it's just climbing the stairs, it all counts. If you take diabetes medication, you can list that, too. The food you eat interacts with the pills or insulin and with exercise, so put that in your record, too.

*W*hat about very-low-calorie diets—
are they recommended for people with
diabetes?

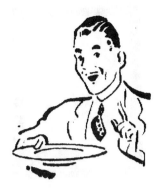

▼
TIP:

Very-low-calorie diets (VLCDs), with less than 800 calories a
day, have been used in the treatment of high-risk overweight
patients and, in particular, people with type 2 diabetes. On this
weight loss program, you drink at least 5 servings of a commercial
formula product daily plus generous amounts of calorie-free beverages, and perhaps some very low calorie food such as lettuce. The
formula has vitamins and minerals to meet the recommended dietary
allowances, because when you eat less than 1,200 calories, you cannot meet your nutritional needs from food alone. Many VLCDs do
not include regular foods that you could buy in the grocery store.
VLCDs appear to be safe if you are evaluated beforehand and
closely monitored by medical professionals. VLCDs produce
significant weight losses and improve your blood glucose levels,
cholesterol, and blood pressure. Unfortunately, using a VLCD alone,
without a behavior-change program, means you probably won't be
able to maintain the weight loss. Some studies report that 5 years
later, most people had maintained only 5% of the amount of weight
they initially lost. More recent reports, however, show that weight
maintenance after a VLCD program is improving. If you have a
strong lifestyle-change program that emphasizes calorie balancing
with increased physical activity, reducing fat calories, and keeping
records, you can keep the weight off. It is important to continue to
have contact with the medical professionals to improve your long-
term maintenance of weight loss, too.

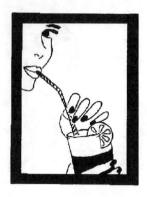

What is a meal replacement?

▼
TIP:

A meal replacement is a portion-controlled food or drink containing 100–300 calories and is used to replace a meal or snack to reduce total calories to lose weight. Meal replacements may be shakes, soups, prepackaged entrees, or snack bars. Meal replacements can be eaten instead of higher-calorie foods. They meet the demands of today's lifestyles for quick and easy dining, while avoiding high-fat, high-calorie choices from fast food chains. Only use meal replacements along with generous serving of fruits and vegetables daily, such as a fruit smoothie with a shake product or one entree plus 2 cups of vegetables. Snack bars offer convenience and variety, and most people like them.

	Calories	Nutrition Value
Formula Shake (one serving)	100–300	1 serving carb 1–2 oz. protein trace fat
Entrees (one)	200–300	2–3 oz. protein 2–3 servings carb less than 5 g fat
Snack Bar (one)	125–250	1 oz. protein 1–2 servings carb less than 5 g fat

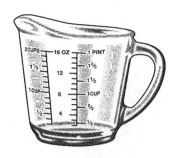

*W*hat are the benefits of using meal replacements?

▼
TIP:

People who use them have significantly greater weight loss than people using standard low-calorie diets. The calorie content is consistent and accurate, so if you use meal replacements, it's easier to reduce your calorie and fat intake and your blood sugar levels if you have diabetes. They are easy to purchase, usually cost less than the meal they replace, are easy to store, and require little or no preparation. They simplify your food choices and help you avoid foods you might overeat. Most weight loss programs that use meal replacements recommend you replace 2 meals and 1 snack a day to lose weight. Replace 1 meal and 1 snack a day to maintain weight.

	Conventional Meals	Meal Replacements	Calorie Savings
Breakfast	Muffin 500 cal	Shake 100 cal	400 cal
Dinner	Meat, starch, vegetable salad 1,000 cal	Entree and 2 cups veggies 350 cal	650 cal

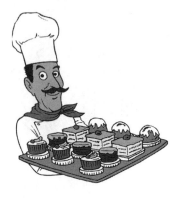

*W*hat are the pitfalls of using meal replacements?

Meal replacements are not for everyone. Some people don't like the taste. If you eat meal replacements in addition to all the other foods you usually eat, you'll take in more calories than usual—and not lose weight. Another problem is overeating meal replacements in the mistaken idea that they are healthy, so eating more is okay. Think of a person who buys a case of 24 snack bars and eats them all in a very short period of time. As you well know, you can get too much of a good thing.

Over time, using meal replacements can become monotonous. You may feel deprived, have food cravings, or start binge eating. Meal replacements should be used only with other healthy foods, especially generous amounts of fruits and vegetables. They were made to help you limit foods that can be problems, such as starchy foods, snack foods, and sweets.

Critics of meal replacement argue that meal replacements are simply a crutch, and do not teach you how to eat foods in the real world. You need to be aware of that to use them correctly.

*H*ow do I select a weight loss
program?

TIP:

*F*irst, decide if you are ready to devote the time, attention, and
effort that is necessary to succeed at weight loss. Then, select
your short-term and long-term weight loss goals. Try to find a
program that will help you meet those goals. Choose a program that
focuses on healthy eating, increased activity, improved self-esteem,
and maintaining the weight loss. Look for programs that help you
change your eating habits through information, guidance, and skills
training. Ask for program literature listing the credentials and training of the staff and factual information about the successful results
of the program, not just personal stories. A safe and sound program
will inform you about any possible risks of the program (especially
if it includes very-low-calorie diets, medications, or surgery). It
should monitor your weight and continue to work with you on your
meal plan and activity habits over time. Discuss with your health
care provider how the program will work for you in light of your
medical history and weight loss expectations. Make a plan for
regular checkups to measure the changes in your health after you
begin the program.

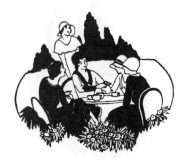

*O*nce I start losing weight, I seem to sabotage myself. What can I do about this pattern?

▼
TIP:

First, identify the ways that you might be sabotaging yourself. Evaluate both your food environment and the way you think about food and dieting. Is your food environment set up for success or sabotage? (See page 104.) If the way you think about food and dieting is sabotaging you, then it is important to change your thoughts and attitudes about eating and losing weight.

1. Try to become aware of any negative thoughts that may set you up for failure.
2. Evaluate these thoughts. Do they make sense? Are they logical, reasonable, or helpful to your goals?
3. If your thoughts do not make sense or are not helpful, try challenging these sabotaging thoughts and substitute a more helpful positive message to think to yourself.
4. Set realistic goals for yourself, so that you are more likely to succeed and have positive thoughts. Give yourself permission to fail. It is unrealistic to think that you can meet all of your goals 100% of the time. If you meet your goals most of the time, you will see progress. Tell yourself that you can do it. Speak well of yourself.

*C*ould skipping breakfast help
me lose weight?

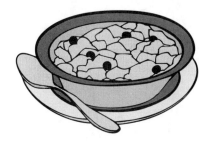

No. You may think you are saving calories by not eating breakfast, but what you are really doing is depriving yourself of a steady supply of glucose, which is your energy source, and setting yourself up for a pattern of overeating at night. If you distribute your meals and snacks evenly throughout the day, you are more likely to avoid periods of over-hunger and overeating. If you have diabetes, this helps you have better blood glucose control.

Ask yourself why you aren't hungry in the mornings. Some people eat so many of their daily calories at supper and in the evening as snacks that even the next morning they still don't feel hungry. This pattern of eating provides your body with a large supply of glucose just in time to go to sleep. If you have diabetes, it can also cause a pattern of high blood sugars overnight. Some people are just not hungry early in the morning. This doesn't mean that you need to skip breakfast. You might be able to eat a small breakfast later if you are not very hungry.

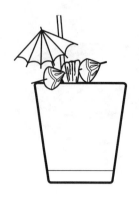

*W*hat effect does alcohol have on weight loss?

▼
TIP:

Alcohol has 7 calories per gram and is metabolized like fat. It has no vitamins or minerals, so those are "empty" calories. Many alcoholic beverages contain calories from sugar, carbohydrate, or fat. Alcohol can also reduce your self-control, leading to overeating. If you have diabetes, alcohol can contribute to problems with hypoglycemia (too low blood glucose). So, if you have diabetes and are on insulin or medications that can cause hypoglycemia, eat a meal or snack with the alcohol to prevent hypoglycemia. All of these factors can lead to too many calories and slow down your weight loss or contribute to weight gain. If you are trying to lose weight by reducing your food intake, it is better to choose foods that are a good source of vitamins and minerals and not the "empty" calories from alcohol. The lowest calorie alcoholic beverages are a 12 oz light beer, 1 oz liquor mixed with diet soda or water, or 5 oz of wine—each contain about 100 calories. Some of the highest calorie alcoholic beverages are made with cream. A 6 oz serving of a White Russian or a Grasshopper contains 450–500 calories. If you also have snacks or extra food with the alcohol, it is easy to see why alcohol can make it more difficult to lose weight!

*H*ow *do I know how many calories to eat each day to lose weight?*

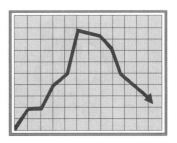

▼
TIP:

The number of calories to eat each day depends on your starting weight and the amount of weight you want to lose each week. Experts recommend a weight loss of 1–2 pounds each week. The chart below lists the number of daily calories to lose 1 pound per week and 2 pounds per week. Don't go below 1,200 calories. You do not need to eat exactly the same number of calories each day. For example, you weigh 210 pounds, so you could start with 1,300–1,500 calories per day to lose 2 pounds per week or 1,800–2,000 calories to lose 1 pound per week. You might decide to be more flexible and let your calories range between 1,300–2,000 calories each day, realizing that on some days you will consume closer to 1,300 calories and on other days, 1,800–2,000 may be more realistic.

Suggested Calorie Goals for Weight Loss

Your current weight (lb)	To lose 1 lb/week	To lose 2 lb/week
Less than 150	1,200 calories*	Not advised
150–200	1,400–1,600 calories	1,200 calories
More than 200	1,800–2,000 calories	1,300–1,500 calories

*If you don't lose weight at this level, it is better to increase your physical activity, than to reduce your calories too much.
Wylie-Rosett et al. *The Complete Weight Loss Workbook,* American Diabetes Association, 1997.

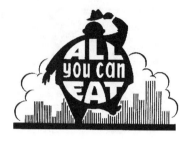

I always feel hungry. Can that really be true?

▼ TIP:

Yes, but it may not necessarily be hunger that you are feeling. You need to learn to distinguish between hunger and appetite. Hunger is a physiological response to the lack of food, and appetite is the desire to eat. Many things can trigger the desire to eat—even when you've just eaten. You can become easily conditioned to think of the desire to eat as hunger. If you find yourself feeling hungry but fairly picky about what you want to eat, ask yourself if it is truly hunger that you are feeling. On the other hand, if you try to cut calories by skipping meals, you are going to feel hungry. Unfortunately your appetite may be so great that it will be difficult to control how much you eat to satisfy that hunger.

If you go on a very-low-calorie diet of less than 1,000 calories, you will feel very hungry much of the time. It is better for you to eat more calories—say 1,200 to 1,500 calories—for a slower but long-term weight loss. In the long run, severely restricting your calories can backfire if you are hungry all the time. And you still have to learn to eat at a higher calorie level to maintain your weight.

Chapter 3
MAINTAINING
YOUR WEIGHT

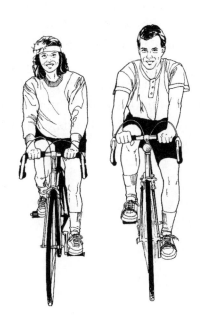

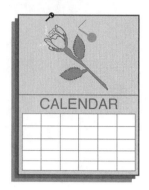

CALENDAR

What is "significant" long-term weight loss?

▼
TIP:

The National Academy of Sciences defines significant weight loss as 5% or more of your initial body weight. This is the amount of weight loss necessary to improve your health—to lower blood glucose and blood pressure and improve cholesterol levels. In practical terms, you might aim for a weight loss of 10% of your body weight to actually achieve a 5–7% weight loss. Another method to express significant weight loss is as a reduction of your BMI by one of more points. Long term means one year or more. For example, a person who weighs 200 pounds, who loses 5–10% of their body weight, would lose 10–20 pounds. A reasonable time-line for reducing body weight by 10% is 6 months, using a reduced-calorie diet. (See page 14.)

*I*s anyone successful with maintaining
weight loss over the long term?

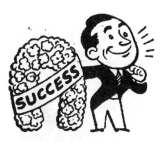

▼
TIP:

Yes, even though maintaining weight loss is the most difficult
part of the process. Research study results have been disap-
pointing, but be careful whose statistics you use. Health care professionals often cite a statistic from 1959, which reports that of those
who manage to lose weight, 95% will regain all of the weight lost.
While we acknowledge the difficulties of weight maintenance, we
KNOW there are individuals who are successful. And the number is
growing. One problem with statistics is that since research typically
reports group averages, the success of individual patients is often
lost in the data. To capture data on successful weight maintenance,
The National Weight Loss Registry was created in 1993 by two
well-known and -respected obesity researchers, Rena Wing, PhD,
at Brown University and Jim Hill, PhD, of Colorado Health
Sciences Center in Denver. The Registry now includes more than
3,000 people who have maintained at least a 30-pound weight loss
for one year or more. In fact, the average person in the Registry has
lost an average of 60 pounds and kept it off for an average of five
and a half years. Yes, you can do it, too.

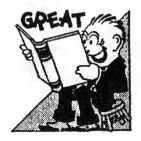

*W*hat are we learning from participants
in the National Weight Loss Registry?

▼
TIP:

The majority (89%) of participants in the Registry report using a combination of diet and physical activity, while 10% use diet alone. One half of them were enrolled in commercial weight loss programs or were under the guidance of a dietitian or psychologist, and half reported losing weight on their own. Of particular interest is that there were no striking differences between how people lost weight and how they were maintaining their weight. The most common method to regulate food intake was to avoid eating certain foods. Most reported eating smaller servings of foods. While they reported a variety of meal planning methods, the most frequently used was counting calories. Most of them report eating less than 30% of daily calories from fat, while some eat less than 20% of calories from fat. Other behaviors that help them succeed are:

- eating an average of 5 small meals per day
- eating breakfast daily
- eating out 3 or fewer meals a week
- weighing themselves regularly, at least once a week
- writing food records
- daily physical activity

H *ow can I predict if I will be able to maintain my weight loss long term?*

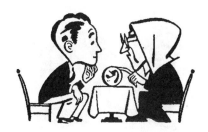

▼
TIP:

O f course, you are an individual and can succeed at maintaining the weight loss on your own. However, research has shown that it helps to participate in a structured program with frequent attendance—weekly or monthly—and if you do, you are likely to be more successful than those who have no follow-up program. We're not sure why so many people regain weight after weight loss. The answers are not simple. Keeping weight off—given the abundance of food, especially high-fat foods, and the limited opportunities for physical activity in the average American's lifestyle—is very difficult. Research supports the following positive and negative predictors of weight maintenance success:

Positive Predictors	Negative Predictors
Physical activity	Negative life events
Record keeping	Family dysfunction
Positive problem-solving attitude	
Continued contact with support	
Normal eating patterns	
Reduction of other health problems (page 49)	

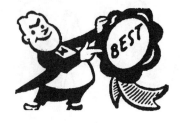

Are there words of encouragement to help me get started and to keep me going on my weight management?

▼
TIP:

Ann Fletcher, RD, has authored two books about "masters of success" with weight loss. She has interviewed hundreds of people who have successfully kept off at least 30 pounds for one year or more. In fact, the people featured in her books have kept off an average of 64 pounds. The average length of time they have kept off 20 (or more) pounds is more than 10 years. Her books tell very familiar stories of people who have struggled with their weight, and then reached a critical point where they finally believed in their own abilities to solve their problems, and how they are now managing successfully. The first volume, *Thin for Life,* is set up according to chapters that discuss ten "keys to success" used by the people interviewed. The second book, *Eating Thin for Life,* includes "food secrets" from the masters, and their favorite recipes. These books are easy reading and very encouraging for your efforts. They are much like the now-famous *Chicken Soup* series for the person who struggles with his weight.

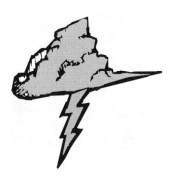

In the National Weight Loss Registry, what "trigger" got patients to start a weight loss program?

▼
TIP:

Most of the participants (77%) said their successful weight loss was triggered by certain dramatic events in their lives. The top three types of triggers were medical problems, emotional events ("my husband left me because I was fat"), and lifestyle events, such as an anniversary or wedding. Men were more likely to say they were losing weight in response to a medical event or simply for the sake of doing it, while women were more likely to cite an emotional or lifestyle event. However, no single reason was given by more than a third of the people. Each person has to find their own trigger. Many times these triggers were unplanned life events, but the important thing is to use the event as an opportunity to get started with lifestyle change.

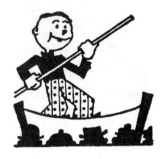

Why do so many people lose weight only to gain it back?

TIP:

Recently it was discovered that genetic factors and complex biochemical systems tend to maintain body weight or return you to the weight you once were. These findings have led to the idea of obesity as a chronic disease rather than a problem simply of overeating, sedentary lifestyle, and lack of willpower. As such, obesity requires lifelong treatment, as with other chronic diseases. Once you have struggled with your weight, you will likely always feel a struggle. To succeed at weight loss and weight maintenance people probably need to see their practitioners more often and over the long term. Since weight management is a skill, it requires time and experience, and a great deal of practice, to develop new behaviors into skills. Unfortunately, many patients are not offered a program to help them maintain weight loss, or they choose not to participate in one. If such a program is offered, take it. Also ask about successful patients who have participated in a maintenance program.

*H*ow *often should I weigh myself?*

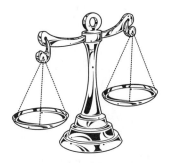

Y ou need to weigh often enough to keep motivated while you are trying to lose weight. For most people weighing once a week is enough to see progress while avoiding playing "games" with the scale. Choose one day of the week and a time for weighing. Keep a log of your weekly weights. You can graph your progress over time.

It is tempting to weigh yourself one or more times a day, but don't. Your weight fluctuates with the amount of water in your system. When you weigh too often, you can convince yourself that you gained more weight eating a big salad and a drinking a 20-oz glass of water than eating a few high-calorie extras. The salad and 20-oz serving of water may show up as a pound or two on the scale, but that weight will be water not body fat. You need to eat 500 calories extra every day to gain a pound every week.

After you get to your weight goal, monitor your weight. Set a 2–5 pound weight cushion. When your weight creeps up by 2 pounds, it's like the yellow traffic signal. Time to monitor your food intake and physical activity more closely and go back to the strategies that helped you lose weight.

Chapter 4
HIGH RISK STAGES OF LIFE

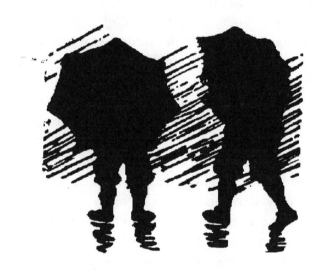

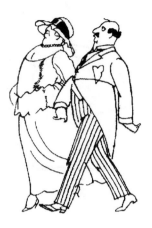

A re you supposed to weigh more as you
reach middle age?

▼
TIP:

Most people gain about 20 pounds or about one pound per year between 25 and 50 years of age. It's not that you're supposed to, but people do. They get less daily physical activity but may eat a little more as they get older. If you eat just 100 extra calories a day, you would eat 35,000 extra calories in a year and gain 10 pounds. Unfortunately, your metabolic rate also slows down as you age, so you don't burn those extra calories. The best plan to fight middle-aged spread is to eat healthfully and to get plenty of activity. Good posture and abdominal exercises may help you feel better, but they do not reduce the health risk associated with abdominal fat. Unfortunately, much of middle-aged weight gain is abdominal fat. You may increase your waist size even if your weight does not change. Having more abdominal fat is associated with health risks such as a rise in blood pressure, triglyceride levels, insulin resistance, and diabetes (page 11). That's a vicious cycle you can stop by getting back to a younger, healthier weight for you.

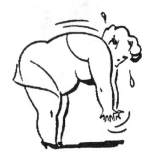

*W*hat effect does menopause have on weight gain?

Both men and women go through midlife hormonal changes. In men, this is called andropause. Weight gain is common during the years of menopause and andropause; however, the reasons for the weight gain do not appear to be due to just the hormones. The body's metabolism slows down as we age because we lose muscle mass, which burns calories. People tend to become less active as they get older, which means we lose muscle mass and burn fewer calories each day. In addition, midlife is also a time when changes in lifestyle, mood, or health can occur, which may affect your eating habits and activity level. The average weight gain is 1 pound a year from age 25 to 55 (or 30 pounds). Hormone changes are associated with changes in body fat distribution and may lead to more fat in the abdomen (page 11). So, even if you are eating the same number of calories each day, you might gain weight if you do not maintain or increase your activity level to preserve your muscle mass and burn extra calories. The bottom line is that if you eat less and increase your activity level, you can lose weight no matter what stage of life you're in.

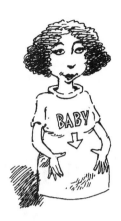

*H*ow does having children affect weight gain
for women?

TIP:

Many women add extra pounds because they do not lose the
weight they gained after having their children. But having
children does not necessarily mean extra weight after delivery.
Women who gain the recommended level of weight during pregnancy have less chance of having a weight problem later. Breast-
feeding helps women return to their normal body weight, too. Many
women want to lose weight during their childbearing years, but few
women make lifestyle changes to accomplish it. Women with young
children need to find a way to focus on their health and weight.
They may need to find a gym that offers programs for young
children during adult exercise classes. There may be parent/child
exercise programs. Being a "soccer mom" can leave little time for
a "mom" exercise program. But you can walk around the soccer
field while you're waiting for the kids. Be aware that buying quanti-
ties of snack foods and eating on the run can put the whole family
at risk for weight gain. Keeping raw fruits and vegetables cut up
and ready to eat for snacks can make it easier for you all to eat
more healthfully.

Chapter 5
WHEN YOU HAVE DIABETES

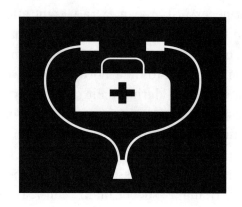

*W*hat are the health benefits of physical
    activity for people with diabetes?

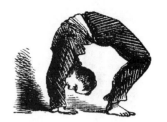

▼
TIP:

B etter blood glucose control! Physical activity burns calories and
lowers your blood glucose. It promotes weight loss, which lowers your blood glucose. Including physical activity in your weight
management program helps you keep muscle while you lose fat,
and muscle burns calories, even at rest—which lowers your blood
glucose. Diabetes puts you at a much higher risk for heart disease.
Exercise improves the health of your heart by keeping it strong and
reducing your waist-to-hip ratio (and abdominal fat). Exercise also
lowers your triglycerides level and raises your high density lipo-
protein (HDL-good) cholesterol level.

Physical activity also has powerful psychological benefits, such
as improved mood, enhanced self-esteem, and a true sense of well-
being. It's the best way to relieve stress. Yes, this lowers blood
glucose levels, too. To get the maximum benefits from exercise for
your diabetes (and keep weight off), enjoy physical activity all
through your life.

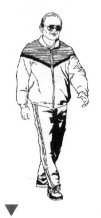

I have a diabetes complication. Is physical activity okay for me to do?

▼
TIP:

A sk your diabetes care team how you can exercise safely. A graded exercise stress test is recommended if you have had type 2 diabetes more than 10 years or are older than 35. Check the following table for more about exercise and diabetes complications.

Exercising Safely with Diabetes Complications

Diabetes Complication	Caution!	Beneficial Activities
Peripheral vascular disease	High impact activities	Moderate walking (may do intermittent exercise with periods of walking followed by periods of rest), non-weight bearing exercise: swimming, cycling, chair exercises
Osteoporosis or arthritis	High impact activities	Moderate daily activities, walking, water exercise, resistance exercise (e.g. light lifting activities), stretching

Hayes, C. *The "I Hate to Exercise" Book,* American Diabetes Association, 2001.

Exercising Safely with Diabetes Complications

Diabetes Complication	Caution!	Beneficial Activities
Heart disease	Very strenuous activity	Moderate activity such as walking, daily chores, gardening, fishing
	Heavy lifting or straining, isometric exercises	Moderate lifting, stretching
	Exercise in extreme heat or cold	Activity in a moderate climate
High blood pressure	Very strenuous activity	Moderate activity such as walking, weight lifting with light weights, stretching
	Heavy lifting or straining and isometric exercise	
Nephropathy (also refer to blood pressure guidelines)	Strenuous activity	Light to moderate daily activities such as walking, light household chores, gardening, water exercise
Neuropathy	Weight bearing activities especially if high impact, strenuous, or prolonged such as: walking a distance, treadmill exercise, step exercise, jumping/ hopping, exercise in heat or cold	Moderate activities that are low impact (e.g. cycling, swimming, chair exercises, stretching), light to moderate daily activities, exercise in a moderate climate
Retinopathy	Strenuous exercise, activities that require heavy lifting and straining, breath holding while lifting or pushing, isometric exercise, high impact activities that cause jarring, head-low activities	Moderate activities that are low impact (e.g. walking, cycling, water exercise), moderate daily chores that do not involve heavy lifting, straining, or the head to be lower than the waist

Hayes, C. The "I Hate to Exercise" Book, American Diabetes Association, 2001.

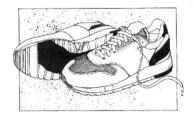

I have neuropathy. What precautions should I take with exercising?

▼
TIP:

If you have neuropathy and loss of feeling in your feet, avoid repetitive weight-bearing exercises, such as long walks or jogging. Try swimming, bicycling, chair exercises, and arm exercises. Never go barefoot except in the bath or bed. You need a good pair of running or walking shoes and socks that wick away moisture. Each time, check your shoes for nails, or pebbles, or tears to the lining before you put them on. Make sure your socks are not too thick for your shoes and that the seam in them is not too thick and putting pressure on your feet. Check your feet after every exercise session for redness, swelling, blisters, or cuts. Get them treated by your doctor promptly.

You should be evaluated regularly for cardiovascular disease. Neuropathy may prevent you from knowing you have it, because you can't feel heart attack pain or pressure. Your blood pressure must be well controlled and monitored. Always do long warm-up and cool-down periods of low intensity before and after each exercise session to ease your heart into and out of the activity.

*W*ill taking diabetes medication make me gain weight?

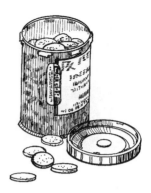

Maybe. When you get better control of your diabetes, you no longer lose glucose in your urine, so your body retains those calories. Some classes of diabetes drugs are more likely to cause weight gain than others. Sulfonylureas (such as glyburide and glipizide), meglitinides (Prandin), and insulin can cause weight gain. The drug class most commonly associated with weight gain and fluid retention is the thiazolidinediones (the glitazones), such as pioglitazone and rosiglitazone. To prevent weight gain, you can intensify your lifestyle efforts (food choices and exercise). The people most likely to develop edema (retain water) are those who already have it. So, women, overweight patients, and those with kidney disease and high blood pressure are at greatest risk. Sometimes doctors prescribe diuretics to control edema and sometimes the patient must switch medications. Metformin works like the glitazones, but doesn't cause weight gain—and may help with weight loss. You can try it instead, being watchful for the side effects of gas, bloating, or diarrhea. You can't take it if you have heart problems. Alpha-glucosidase inhibitors (such as acarbose and miglitol) don't cause weight gain, either, but side effects can be gas, bloating, or diarrhea.

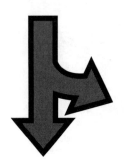

How can I lose weight and not get discouraged by more frequent episodes of hypoglycemia?

TIP:

Any time you reduce the amount of food you eat, your blood sugar will be lower even before the first pound is lost, which is good. Most people with type 2 diabetes won't have a problem with hypoglycemia (blood glucose below 60). But people who take insulin or diabetes pills that can cause hypoglycemia need to monitor their blood sugar levels on a weight loss program. You treat hypoglycemia by eating a snack with 15 grams of carbohydrate, but you don't want to be eating more food than is on your meal plan. Instead, it might work better to lower the dosage of your medication. As you lose weight, watch the trends in your blood sugar patterns and discuss making changes in your doses of insulin or pills with your doctor before your blood sugar levels get too low. Another way to help prevent hypoglycemia as you lose weight is to focus on lowering your fat intake and keeping your carbohydrate intake about the same at the same meal each day. If your carbohydrate intake at meals and snacks varies widely from day to day, then you are more likely to have erratic blood sugars and possibly more hypoglycemia.

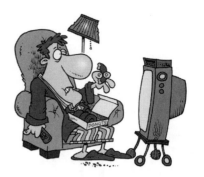

*W*hat are the recommendations
for exercise for people with
diabetes?

▼
TIP:

Do it. You need aerobic exercise and strength training to make
your heart and lungs strong, gain muscles and strength, lower
blood pressure, improve circulation, and lower blood glucose. Blood
sugar is lower for 12–24 hours. How low depends on how long and
how hard you exercise, the blood glucose level before exercise, and
how fit you are. Some people notice higher blood sugar levels after
exercise. This may be caused by hormonal changes in response
to exercise or because blood sugar was high (more than 300)
before exercise in people with type 1 who are not taking enough
insulin. People with type 2 diabetes should exercise at least every
other day and, ideally, most days of the week. This helps control
blood sugar, which could be higher on days that you are sedentary
and lower on days that you are active. Drink water before, during,
and after exercise. It helps you keep going. If hypoglycemia is a
problem for you, instead of eating too many snacks, work with your
health care team to reduce your insulin or diabetes pills, so your
blood sugar won't drop too low (below 70) during or after exercise.
Carry a snack in case you need one.

Chapter 6
PREVENTING DIABETES

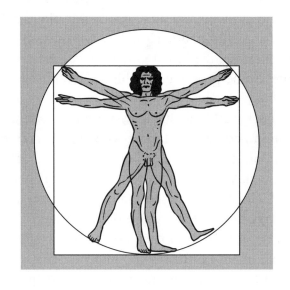

*W*ill losing weight help me
   prevent getting diabetes?

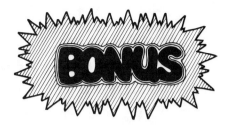

▼
TIP:

Yes, the DPP shows that people with impaired glucose tolerance
(IGT) who lose 10–15 pounds reduce their risk of getting type
2 diabetes by more than 50%. If you are older than 60, the DPP
found that losing this amount of weight reduced the risk of diabetes
by 71%. Good news—these effects were the same for men and
women and all minority groups. In addition, one-third of the people
who lost the weight and exercised at least 150 minutes per week
(30 min × 5 days) improved their blood sugar levels from IGT to
normal. (If you have impaired glucose tolerance, your body isn't
taking the glucose out of your blood as efficiently as it should.)
So, not only does losing weight help prevent diabetes, it also helps
bring blood sugar levels that are above normal back to normal! The
Finnish Diabetes Prevention study had similar results. A weight loss
of 11% of body weight (more than 15 pounds) was associated with
more than an 80% reduction in risk of getting type 2 diabetes. These
results strongly suggest that the more weight you can lose, the better
chance you have of preventing type 2 diabetes.

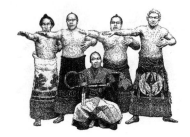

How do I know if I am at risk for diabetes?

▼

TIP:

Some people have diabetes and do not know it. You should be screened every 3 years beginning at age 45 and perhaps, more frequently if you have risk factors for diabetes. The risk increases with age, weight gain, and inactivity. The major risk factors are:

- Family history of diabetes (parents or siblings)
- Overweight (BMI ≥25)
- High blood pressure (≥140/90)
- HDL cholesterol ≤35mg/dl
- Triglyceride level ≥250 mg/dl
- Diabetes during pregnancy or a baby weighing more than 9 lbs
- Polycystic ovary syndrome
- Ethnic groups (African American, Latin American, American Indian, Asian American, Pacific Islanders)

W*hat's the difference between IGT and diabetes?*

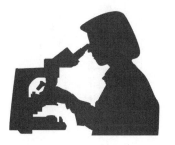

▼
TIP:

The difference is in your blood sugar levels. The most common test for diabetes is a fasting blood sugar level (taken after at least 8 hours without food). If your fasting blood sugar is less than 110, it is normal. You do not have diabetes. If it is 111–125, you have impaired fasting glucose or IFG (pre-diabetes). If it is 126 or greater, then you have diabetes.

Another screen for diabetes is an oral glucose tolerance test. This involves getting a fasting blood sugar test, then drinking a sweetened drink, and getting a second blood sugar test 2 hours later. If the 2-hour blood test is less than 140, it is normal. If it is 141–199, you have IGT, meaning that your body is not using glucose the way it should. This is also called pre-diabetes. If the result is 200 or greater, you have diabetes. To confirm the diagnosis using either of these testing methods, you need to have a second test on another day.

	Normal	Pre-Diabetes	Diabetes
Fasting blood sugar	110	111–125	>126
2-hr blood sugar	140	141–199	>200

When you have pre-diabetes, it may be because you are insulin resistant. Your body may make plenty of insulin but cannot use it correctly, so your glucose levels are too high. Being overweight is one of the causes of insulin resistance.

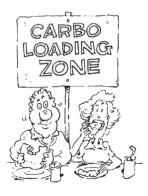

Does insulin resistance lead to weight gain?

▼
TIP:

Scientific evidence suggests that it is being overweight that causes insulin resistance rather than insulin resistance causing weight gain. Most Americans are gaining weight instead of losing because we are eating more total calories (100–300 extra calories per day) and exercising less. Many overweight adults eat too many calories from carbohydrate-rich foods as they try to cut back on fatty foods. If you eat too much carbohydrate and you are insulin resistant, then it will cause higher blood sugar levels as well as contribute extra calories. Too much is too much. To lose weight successfully and reduce insulin resistance, reduce your calories by decreasing the amounts of both carbohydrates and fats that you eat. Any diet with fewer calories than you usually eat will help you lose weight and reduce insulin resistance. The key is to find a pattern of eating that has a healthy balance between all the food groups and is lower in calories than your usual diet.

*D*oes exercise help prevent
diabetes?

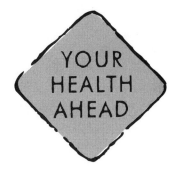
YOUR
HEALTH
AHEAD

▼
TIP:

Yes, research shows that increasing your activity level is an
important lifestyle change for preventing diabetes. In the DPP,
participants in the lifestyle-change group were asked to exercise at
least 150 minutes a week. Most of them chose brisk walking, and
others started swimming or biking. The average activity level was
208 minutes in the first year and 189 minutes at the end of the
3-year study. Another study in China showed that increasing physical activity can reduce the risk of developing diabetes by 46%.
Participants in this study were asked to increase their exercise level
by 2 units (see chart) a day for those over 50 years old who had no
problems with heart disease or arthritis. The average activity level
was 4 units per day. The clear message is that activity alone—even
without weight loss—is a powerful diabetes prevention strategy.

Activities Required for One Unit of Exercise

Intensity	Time (minutes)	Exercise
Mild	30	Slow walking, traveling, shopping, housecleaning
Moderate	20	Faster walking, going downstairs, cycling, doing heavy laundry, ballroom dancing (slow)
Strenuous	10	Slow running, climbing stairs, disco dancing for the elderly, playing volleyball or table tennis
Very strenuous	5	Jumping rope, playing basketball, swimming

The Da Qing IGT and Diabetes study. *Diabetes Care.* 1997; 20(4): 537–544.

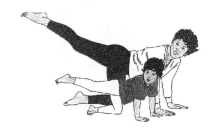

Why are so many teenagers overweight?

Today almost half of the children and teens in the United States are overweight. There has also been a dramatic increase in type 2 diabetes among these children. Environmental changes are the cause of this epidemic of obesity and diabetes. Children are bombarded with food advertising and have fewer opportunities for physical activity than in the past. This is a toxic environment with respect to diabetes risk. Kids who watch too much TV or play computer games for more than 2 hours a day, drink lots of sugared beverages, eat large portions of snack foods, and eat under stress gain lots of weight. The government and volunteer health organizations, including the American Diabetes Association (ADA), are working to reduce obesity through research and public health campaigns to promote healthier habits. Parents and kids need to make some changes: decrease the amount of time watching TV, increase after-school recreation programs, and be more physically active. They need to stop making a daily habit of eating fast foods and drinking sugared beverages. The government is making an effort to change the way foods are packaged and marketed to children, but parents and family members have to help the kids make the changes they need.

Chapter 7
WEIGHT LOSS SURGERY AND MEDICATIONS

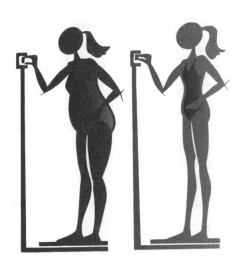

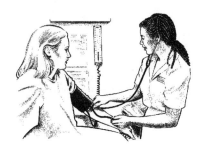

*A re weight loss drugs
beneficial?*

▼
TIP:

Weight loss drugs that have been approved by the Food and Drug Administration (FDA) for long-term use can be beneficial—along with lifestyle changes—for some patients with a BMI of 30 or more but no other health conditions, and for patients with a BMI of 27 or more with health problems. The health problems important enough to justify use of drugs are high blood pressure, high cholesterol, heart disease (CHD), type 2 diabetes, and sleep apnea. Your health must be monitored the whole time you are taking the drug.

At the present time, two drugs are available for long-term use: sibutramine and orlistat. Sibutramine enhances weight loss and can help with weight loss maintenance. Potential side effects with drugs must be kept in mind. With sibutramine, increases in blood pressure and heart rate may occur. So, sibutramine should not be used if you have high blood pressure, heart disease, congestive heart failure, arrhythmias, or a history of stroke. With orlistat, you may need fat-soluble vitamins because you can't absorb them as well. You should be carefully monitored for any side effects.

*S*hould I have surgery to lose weight?

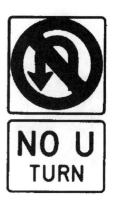

▼
TIP:

M aybe, if you have a BMI of 40 or greater. People with a BMI between 35 and 40 may be considered for surgery if they have medical conditions such as diabetes, high blood pressure, or arthritis and problems moving around. Surgery is considered for people between 18 and 65 years old who have made many unsuccessful attempts to lose weight in supervised programs. The types of weight loss surgery are Vertical Banded Gastroplasty (VBG) and Gastric Bypass (GB). VBG uses stainless steel staples or a plastic "belt" to create a small pouch separate from the rest of the stomach. The pouch holds only a small amount of food, limiting how much you can eat before feeling full. Gastric bypass creates a small pouch and causes food to bypass the first part of the small intestine to reduce food absorption, producing more weight loss than VBG. For both surgeries, there are risks of the pouch stretching and the staples rupturing if you overeat. Gastric bypass has higher risk for nutritional deficiencies and dumping syndrome. (Your stomach contents "dump" too rapidly through the small intestine and cause nausea, weakness, and diarrhea.) Even with surgery, you still need to make lasting lifestyle changes.

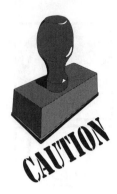

W hat should I consider before having surgery for weight loss?

▼
TIP:

Surgery to lose weight is a serious undertaking. You should clearly understand the benefits and the risks.

Benefits: Most people lose weight rapidly. After the first 6–9 months, the rate of weight loss usually slows down, but some people lose weight for 18–24 months. Weight losses of 60% have been reported 5 years after gastric bypass surgery. This surgery can help control type 2 diabetes without medications, because the weight loss often leads to normal blood sugar levels and also improves, or resolves, other obesity-related health problems such as high blood pressure, high cholesterol, and sleep apnea.

Risks: Approximately 10–20% of people require follow-up surgery to correct complications or side effects. The most common are hernias and vitamin B12 deficiency (corrected with supplements or monthly B12 shots). Serious complications are rupture of the staple line or a stretched stomach pouch caused by overeating. One-third of the patients develop gallstones. Another possible side effect is dumping syndrome. It occurs after eating foods with concentrated sugar and results in sweating, nausea, weakness, abdominal pain, and diarrhea due to the rapid passage of sugars into the small intestine. Dumping syndrome can be managed with attention to your diet. Any surgery under a general anesthetic also carries some risk to the patient's life.

*W*hat happens after weight loss
surgery?

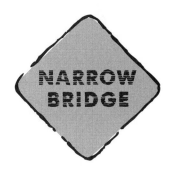

NARROW
BRIDGE

▼
TIP:

Y ou get full faster, and you don't absorb foods as well. This can
cause nausea, abdominal pain, diarrhea, and vomiting if you eat
too much food at once or foods high in fat or sugar. Most people
take 3–6 months to go through the 4 diet stages from no-added-
sugar clear liquids to 3 meals and 1–2 snacks a day. It is common to
have lactose (milk) intolerance and vitamin and mineral deficiencies.
Anemia can result from poor absorption of vitamin B12 and iron in
menstruating women. Decreased calcium absorption may increase
your risk of osteoporosis. You must take iron, calcium, and vitamin
B12 supplements daily for the rest of your life. Some people have
difficulty with certain foods, such as red meat, bread, or pasta. Other
people can eat all foods, including sweets, while others have taste
changes. An experienced health care team must oversee your transi-
tion to whole foods and find the right levels of vitamin and calcium
supplements. If you drink high-calorie beverages and graze on small
portions of food all day, you can gain weight back. You need to take
responsibility for your eating habits for a lifetime if you want to
keep the weight off.

SECTION II
Activity

Chapter 8
THE BASICS

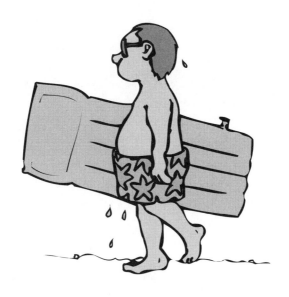

*H*ow can I get started being physically active?

▼
TIP:

C hoose an activity you enjoy to increase the chances you'll stick with it. Walking is most popular and most frequently recommended for overweight people. Start out slowly, walking about 10 minutes 5 days a week. Gradually increase to walking 30 minutes 5 days a week. You can also take the stairs, mow the lawn, and run the vacuum. Most weight loss programs encourage you to do both types of activity to burn the most calories.

You don't need to sweat or join a gym, but having a trainer at the beginning helps you succeed. Keeping records of your physical activity (minutes or calories burned) in your food record helps you identify patterns and provides good feedback on your progress. You'll be able to see the connection between calories burned and weight loss. Measure your hips, waist, biceps, and thighs. Muscle weighs more than fat, so if you don't see a change in the scale, you'll be able to encourage yourself with the changes in your measurements—and how your clothes fit, too!

While you walk, you can listen to tapes that encourage you and help you vary the pace for a better work out. Or you can get a book on tape from the library and enjoy it while you get your exercise.

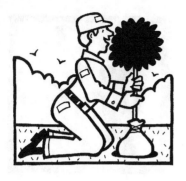

*C*an I increase my physical
activity using everyday
activities?

▼
TIP:

Yes. The Lifetime Activity Model encourages using types of
activity that are already part of your everyday routine activities.
These activities might include vacuuming, mowing the lawn with a
push mower, house painting, car washing, yard work, gardening,
taking the stairs, parking the car further away and walking, and just
walking more. (Get a pedometer!) These activities can be done at
various speeds and for varying lengths of time.

Activity Benefits of Household Chores and Yard Work

Activity Category		Average Calories Burned/ 30 minutes*
Light Household Chores		90 to 100 calories
Cooking/baking	Light carpentry	
Dusting furniture	Sweeping floors	
Laundry	Washing dishes	
Moderate House and Yard Work		130 to 190 calories
Gardening	Carrying out trash	
Mowing the lawn/	or recycling	
hedging and trimming	Vacuuming floors	
Raking leaves	Washing cars	
Scrubbing floors	Washing windows	
Hard House and Yard Work		over 200 calories
Digging light earth	Home repair	
Shoveling snow		

*Calories burned per 30 min are for an individual who weighs 150 pounds. Actual
calories burned are slightly less for people who weigh under 150 pounds and are
slightly more for those who weigh over 150 pounds.
Hayes, C. *The "I Hate to Exercise" Book,* American Diabetes Association, 2001.

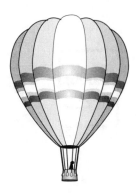

*W*hy do I need to warm up and stretch
before I exercise?

▼
TIP:

The warm-up helps get the blood flowing a little more quickly,
which helps your body prepare for more vigorous work. You
should warm up gradually by walking slowly, doing light calisthen-
ics, or dancing. You want to gradually increase your heart rate to
within 20 beats of your target range (page 75). The warm-up also
gives your muscles and joints a chance to loosen up. End your
warm-up with stretching each part of your body. No single stretch
can take care of your whole body. Begin at your neck and work
down to the ankles. Start with neck rotations, move to shoulder rolls
and arm swings, do a gentle knee bend, and finish with ankle rotations. Stretch the tendons that support your major joints to the point
of tension, but not to the point of pain. Do NOT bounce as you
stretch because it is hard on joints and muscles. Breathe deeply and
relax into the stretch. Each joint and muscle group should be
stretched for 5–30 seconds. You are prepared now to get the full
benefit of your aerobic exercise without injury.

Why do I need to cool down and stretch after I finish exercising?

▼
TIP:

A cool-down helps slow your heart rate down and helps muscles and joints return to an inactive state. You reduce your chances of injury and sore muscles if your brisk walks and other aerobic activities include the warm-up and stretch before you start and cool-down and stretch after you finish. You can slow down your aerobic activity or walk slowly for 5–10 minutes after aerobic activity to cool down. The cool-down should end with stretching. Again the stretching includes neck rotations, shoulder rolls, arm swings, gentle knee bends, and ankle rotations. Your stretches should be smooth, fluid movements. As you do in yoga, you can hold a stretch, but do not make jerky, sudden movements or bounces. After the cool-down and stretching, your body should feel relaxed and more flexible. Your heart rate should have returned to its normal pre-exercise rate by the end of the cool-down and stretch.

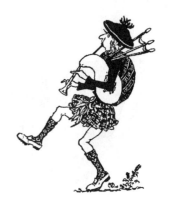

*W*hy do I have leg pains when I walk?

▼
TIP:

Sore muscles can hurt when you walk, but pain can also be a symptom of poor circulation. If you have diabetes or other cardiovascular risk factors such as high blood pressure, your doctor should evaluate the pain. You may have intermittent claudication or poor blood flow. Intermittent claudication feels like cramping or aching. The pain occurs because the blood vessels leading to the lower leg have narrowed, and the muscles cannot get enough blood. The pain usually occurs after you walk a short distance. Your physician may recommend that you walk until you begin to feel pain, stop to rest, and walk some more. You gradually increase the distance walked and improve circulation to your leg, relieving the pain.

Leg pain can also be due to sore muscles. If you are out of condition and try to walk quickly, you may feel discomfort in your legs. You may be stretching muscles that are not used to stretching. If you run or exercise vigorously, you can get shin splints, or tendonitis on the front of the lower leg. Walk more slowly or do a different activity for a few days until the soreness goes away.

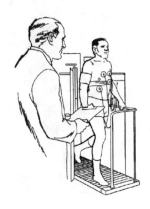

W *hat is a stress test?*

▼
TIP:

T he purpose of an exercise stress test is to find out how much
exercise you can safely do. An exercise stress test may also be
used to develop a cardiac rehabilitation program for people who
have had a heart attack or as a tool for evaluating heart disease. You
may be asked to exercise on a treadmill or on a stationary bike for
the test. Your blood pressure, electrocardiogram (ECG), and heart
rate are measured throughout the test, which usually lasts less than
30 minutes. Exercise stress testing provides a controlled environment for observing the effects of increasing demand for oxygen by
the heart. An ECG can provide evidence of damage to the coronary
arteries that supply blood to the heart muscles. Blood pressure
changes also provide information about the fitness of the heart. If
you have an exercise stress test, you may be asked to report symp-
toms such as fatigue, chest pain, or shortness of breath to provide a
more complete picture of how well your heart functions. A stress
test may tell you your maximum heart rate. You use this to figure
your target heart rate during exercise.

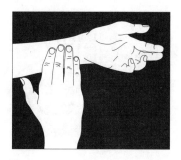

*W*hy should I check my target heart rate?

▼
TIP:

The target heart rate is usually 60–80% of your maximum heart rate (which can be determined by a mathematical formula or a stress test). You need activity levels high enough to increase blood circulation and your heart rate. However, you should not put too much stress on your heart. Your target heart rate keeps you in the safe but effective range. You have probably exceeded your target heart rate if you have difficulty catching your breath or talking while exercising. Consult with your provider if you have diabetes or heart disease. If you take medications such as beta-blockers, your heart rate may not increase with physical activity.

You can take your pulse at the arteries on either side of your windpipe or the artery 1/4 inch inside your wrist below the thumb. Do not use your thumb to take a pulse.

Target Heart Rates for Healthy People

Age	Beats per minute 60%	Beats per minute 80%	Beats/6 seconds range
20	120	160	12–16
30	114	152	11–15
40	108	144	10–14
50	102	136	10–14
60	96	128	9–13
70	90	120	9–12
80	84	112	8–11

Wylie-Rosett et al. *The Complete Weight Loss Workbook,* American Diabetes Association, 1997.

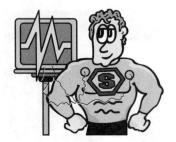

*D*o *I need an exercise stress test?*

▼

TIP:

A sk your physician. You may need an exercise stress test if you are increasing the intensity of physical activity. If you have diabetes or heart disease, you may need a stress test. In addition to being used in cardiac programs, exercise stress tests are often used as part of fitness planning. If you join a fitness center, you may need an exercise stress test to make sure that you can safely participate in various activities and to help you set exercise goals.

Good Reasons to Consult Your Physician before Beginning Exercise

---

- You are a male over age 40 or a female over age 50
- You have diabetes and are over age 35
- You have had type 2 diabetes for more than 10 years
- You have had type 1 diabetes for more than 15 years
- You have high blood triglycerides, high blood cholesterol, or low HDL cholesterol
- You have heart disease
- You have high blood pressure
- You take heart or blood pressure medications
- You have retinopathy, nephropathy, or autonomic neuropathy
- You have experienced chest pain or pressure, faintness, or dizziness

---

*W*hy *do you recommend walking and step counters?*

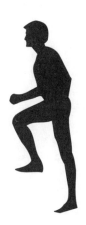

▼
TIP:

Walking is inexpensive, easy, and convenient. More than 60% of adults in the United States get less than the recommended level of physical activity of 30 minutes 5 days a week. Inactive people take an average of 2,000 to 4,000 steps per day. Moderately active people take 5,000 to 7,000 steps per day. Active people take at least 10,000 steps per day. People who have diabetes are more likely to be inactive than other people. High blood sugars can make you feel tired and sluggish, so you don't exercise. But, studies have shown that a walking program can increase your insulin sensitivity for up to 72 hours—lowering blood sugar and giving you more energy.

Pedometers can help you count (and increase) the number of steps you take each day. You can purchase an inexpensive pedometer in most stores with sporting goods. Slightly more expensive pedometers measure distance as well. You can estimate the distance from your number of steps. Walking 2,000 steps is about one mile. Awareness of the number of steps helps you think of creative ways to take more. You can even purchase a "talking" pedometer to boost your motivation while you walk.

SECTION III
Variety

Chapter 9
PLANNING FOR SUCCESS

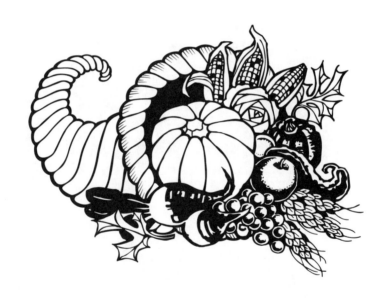

*A*t *a certain point my weight gets stuck at a plateau. What can I do when the scale won't budge?*

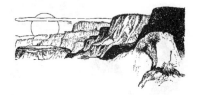

TIP:

When this happens, ask yourself some questions:

1. Am I keeping track of calories and fat grams?
2. Are my serving sizes correct? Am I eyeballing portions, or actually weighing and measuring to be sure they are correct?
3. Based on my current weight, do I need to reduce my calories to continue to lose weight?
4. Have I been active enough?

If you answer "no" to any of these questions, you have a possible cause of the plateau. If you answer "yes" to all of the questions, take a look at your weight loss pattern over time. Not everyone loses the same amount each week. Some people lose 2–4 pounds in one week and then don't lose any weight for 2 weeks despite healthy eating and activity. Other people retain fluid from time to time that masks their true body weight. If you know that your eating habits and activity are on target, then weight loss will usually follow. The key is to find ways to stay motivated while the plateau lasts. Find other ways to chart your progress, such as measuring your waist or thigh with a tape measure, so you can see the inches you've lost.

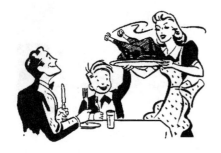

*H*ow can I deal with vacations and holidays so I don't regain weight?

▼
TIP:

Vacations and holidays are the times when most people let go and enjoy food and relaxation. So you need to set reasonable goals for your weight and activity. It may be more reasonable to expect to maintain your weight rather than lose any during vacations. Resume weight loss once the holiday is over. Plan ahead for eating out. You might decide to limit the number of times you eat out and spend the extra time and money on other activities. When you go out, eat what you want, but you can limit calories by eating smaller servings. Set up your food environment for success by bringing low-calorie food choices with you. Think ahead about what you might like to do to stay active. Before you go, discuss your eating and activity goals with family and friends and ways that they can support you. If you plan, you are more likely to meet your goals. But remember it takes 3 or 4 holidays before you get the plan just right. Learn from your experiences. See what helped you and what stopped you. Adjust your strategy the next time. Don't get discouraged, be patient, and keep trying!

How can I learn to manage binge eating, so I can succeed with weight loss?

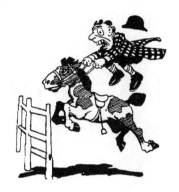

▼
TIP:

Binge eating is overeating that feels out of control. Binge eating is associated with higher body weight, more difficulty losing weight, and higher blood sugar levels. If you want to manage problems with binge eating, the first step is to keep food records. Then you can clearly see your patterns with binge eating and how they change as you try different strategies. Look at your food records to find:

- What you eat during binges (forbidden foods?)
- When binges occur (evenings, weekends, weekdays?)
- Triggers for binges (emotions, stress, loneliness?)
- Reasons for binges (to relieve tension, distract from problems?)

It is also important to check your weight once a week around the same time of day to evaluate your weight trends over time. Once you have a system to track your eating patterns and weight trends, then you are ready to try out different strategies to manage binge eating. As you try a strategy, check your food records for changes in the number of binge eating episodes, the types of food that you eat, the timing of binges, the triggers for binges, and the functions that binges serve.

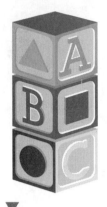

What strategies can I try to reduce binge eating?

TIP:

Some of the strategies to manage binge eating are:

1. Keep food records.
2. Establish a regular pattern of eating with 3 meals and 2–3 snacks. Do not skip meals.
3. Eat every 3–4 hours. Most people binge when they are either over-hungry or have too much free time.
4. If you eat or binge between planned meals and snacks, go right back to your regular pattern as quickly as possible.
5. Eat more slowly and focus on savoring each bite. Enjoy the sight, the smell, the taste, and the texture of your food. It is easier to do this if you sit down, and you don't watch TV, read, or work while eating.
6. Rearrange your food environment (page 109).
7. Rearrange your emotional environment (page 114).
8. Make a list of activities you enjoy that help distract you from the urge to binge or make it difficult to binge (exercise, visit friends, work on a hobby).

Remember it takes time, patience, and practice to find the combination of strategies that works best for you.

*H*ow do I know if a slip from healthy
eating is a problem or not?

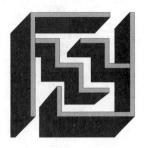

▼
TIP:

E veryone who is trying to eat healthy to lose weight is going to
slip. Some people call it cheating, but it's okay. It's normal. It is
usually not the slip that is the problem, rather it is the way we react
to slips when they happen. The truth is that no one slip can ruin
your overall progress. Slips are part of the process of changing your
eating habits. One slip is not a pattern. However, if you notice a
series of slips and that you are returning to old habits, losing your
overall focus, and have gained back more than 3 pounds, then take
steps to refocus and seek help. Try to make a list of the "clues" that
show you are dealing with more than just a slip. For example, clues
on your list might include a weight gain of more than 3 pounds,
more than one week without exercising, certain clothes are too tight,
or an old habit that you had worked hard to break comes back.

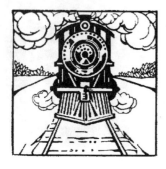

*O*nce I slip from healthy eating and gain weight, how can I get back on track?

▼
TIP:

We learn from mistakes, so they are valuable. Make sure your reaction to slips or cheating on your diet doesn't work against you.

1. Don't engage in negative self-talk or blame. Talk positively to yourself and *about* yourself. Instead of thinking "I blew it," try thinking "One slip won't ruin everything. I can get back to eating better right now." Your positive thoughts affect how you feel and what you do.
2. Look for why the slip happened and try to learn from the experience. Everyone who tries to eat healthy and lose weight has their own list of high-risk situations that cause slips. This is your chance to learn more about the situations that put you at high risk. Then you can think about how to avoid a slip the next time.
3. Talk to someone. Family, friends, co-workers, and others can be a real source of support. Talk about what caused you to slip, what you have learned from the situation, and your ideas for handling this high-risk situation in the future. Consider regular appointments with a dietitian or counselor for more professional help.

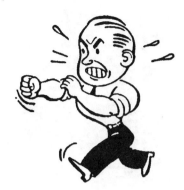

I *know how to lose weight, but how do
I get the willpower to do it?*

Willpower is the ability to resist eating tempting foods in your environment. If you rely only on willpower for success with weight loss, your success will probably be short-lived because the motivation to resist eating tempting foods can wax and wane over time. To lose weight you learn the best food choices, but you also shift away from relying on willpower to making a habit of self-control. You build self-control when you rearrange your food environment and change the way you think about food and dieting, so your desire to eat arises less frequently and less intensely.

There are several ways to rearrange your food environment for success.

1. Keep away from problem foods by not buying them or putting them out of sight.
2. Keep a variety of healthy low-calorie food choices around you.
3. Don't go long periods (more than 4–5 hours) without food, as this can lead to over-hunger, food cravings, and a greater tendency to overeat.
4. Choose lower-calorie foods.
5. Engage in activities away from food.

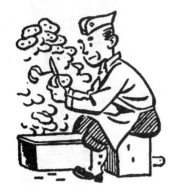

I get bored eating the same foods, and crave foods I shouldn't eat. How can I manage this problem?

▼ TIP:

You need to introduce new healthy foods into meals and maybe change the times you eat, too. Mix it up. Variety is important. When you notice you are feeling bored, ask:

- Do I sacrifice variety for convenience or speed in the lunches I carry or the dinners I make? What other foods could I use?
- What meals, snacks, or foods am I most bored with?
- How can I vary this part of my eating and still lose weight?
- Would changes in taste, texture, or temperature make my meals more satisfying and interesting? Do I want something spicy, instead of sweet or bland? Something hot, cold, or at room temperature? Something crunchy, chewy, or smooth?

When you answer the questions, you see ways to vary meals and snacks, so you are not bored or craving unhealthy foods. At the library, you can search food magazines and healthy cookbooks for quick meal recipes and new foods to meet your personal needs for taste, texture, and temperature. Have fun with your meal plan. It's one of the most important things you do each day.

*S*hould I take vitamin supplements *while I'm cutting back on food to lose weight?*

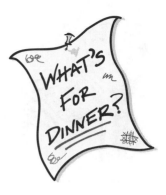

▼
TIP:

If you cut back on food to lose weight and you're not eating a healthy diet as described in the Food Guide Pyramid, then you may need a multivitamin supplement. The Food Guide Pyramid recommends eating a variety of foods and a daily minimum of:

- 6 servings of bread, cereal, rice, or pasta (a serving is usually 1 slice or 1/2 cup)
- 3 servings of vegetables
- 2 servings of fruit
- 2 servings of dairy (milk, yogurt, or cheese)
- 2 servings of meat, fish, poultry, eggs, legumes

If your diet does not include this number of servings from each of these food groups, then it is possible that you are not getting enough protein or the vitamins and minerals that you need. A registered dietitian can help you determine the nutritional quality of your diet and tell you if it is lacking any vitamins or minerals.

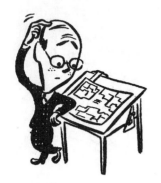

*H*ow does food combining really work?

Several popular weight loss diets recommend avoiding specific combinations of foods to improve digestion and metabolism. They say that starchy foods are to be eaten alone to improve weight loss. People who go on these diets often do lose weight, but it's because they eat fewer calories. The food combining approach encourages people to eat a lot of fruits and vegetables, a modest amount of starches, and limited portions of meat. This is okay, but milk and dairy foods are not permitted at all. Each type of food is basically eaten alone, which reduces the tendency to overeat. This structured approach does help avoid the added calories that come from unplanned eating. But you need very careful timing and planning to allow the recommended time before eating a food that should not be combined with a previously eaten food. The dietary plan tends to be low in calcium, vitamin B12, Vitamin D, zinc, and protein.

*D*oes grapefruit help you burn fat and lose weight?

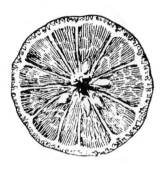

The answers are "No" to fat burning, but "Yes" to helping you lose weight. Many popular weight loss diets promote grapefruit with claims that the acid in the grapefruit will burn fat. And people who ritualistically eat grapefruit before their meals are likely to lose weight. The reason is that grapefruit is filling and relatively low in calories, so you are likely to be satisfied with less food when you eat the meal.

There are no research studies that support the claim that grapefruit burns body fat, speeds up metabolism, or causes weight loss by any other type of miracle. While grapefruit is not a miracle food for burning fat, it is a great option for filling up on more wholesome foods. The bottom line is that you may find eating grapefruit helpful, but you have to do more than just eat grapefruit to lose weight.

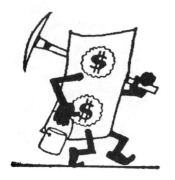

Diet food and all those fruits and vegetables seem so expensive. How can following my meal plan cost less?

▼ TIP:

You can budget money as you are budgeting calories. You do not need to buy high-priced diet foods. Fresh vegetables and fruit and foods that you prepare yourself are always the less expensive choice. You can choose to spend some time and save some money.

Low-calorie frozen entrées tend to cost more than the regular versions. Ones that have more meat cost more than the pasta-based frozen entrees. Cutting down on high-priced meat can help save money that you can use to buy vegetables and fruits. Store brands of frozen vegetables are usually lower priced than national brands. When buying vegetables, compare the bagged ones with the ones you buy by the pound. Buying fruits in season can help save money—apples in the fall, citrus fruits in the winter, and berries in the spring. Another way to save money is to buy produce directly from the farmer. The web site for the United States Department of Agriculture *www.nal.usda.gov/afsic/csa/* provides information about the Community Supported Agriculture (CSA) program, which links local farmers to consumer buying groups whose members buy a share of the weekly harvest during the growing season.

*D*oes drinking water help you lose weight?

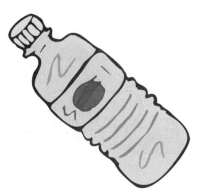

▼
TIP:

Yes, drinking water can help you lose weight. Water contains no calories, and it helps you feel full. Experts recommend that we drink 8 glasses of water a day for good health. A growing number of weight- and health-conscious people have increased their daily water intake by carrying a bottle of water with them wherever they go.

Unfortunately, many people drink too many soft drinks instead of water. The obesity epidemic in our country is linked to the popularity of drinking bigger sizes of sugar-rich sports drinks and soft drinks. If you drink these instead of water, you should know that a 20-oz soft drink contains 300–400 calories and 15–20 teaspoons of sugar. That is 12–15 calories per ounce. Fruit juices also contain 12 calories per ounce. Even the sports drinks are 6–10 calories per ounce. These calorie levels make water a very attractive option, indeed. If you are not a fan of water, consider seltzer (without added sugar). Diet soft drinks are another option, but for health and variety, drink water, too.

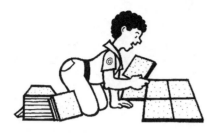

*C*an I just make up my own diet?

▼
TIP:

Yes. Start with the foods you like, your daily schedule, and your health needs. You can use the food pyramid or exchanges or carbohydrate counts in the meal plan.

1. **Limit choices.** For most people, as the variety of food increases, the amount of food eaten and calories also increase. Consider not keeping tempting foods at home and what to do when eating out. You might try some meal replacements (page 24).
2. **Identify and change behaviors leading to too many calories.** Some people don't eat all day and have an uncontrolled appetite at night. Eat breakfast, lunch, and dinner. For other people, simply eating fewer sugared beverages or snack foods makes a big difference.
3. **Become aware of your eating.** Many people are unaware of what or how much they eat. Learn more about your eating style. Slow down and chew each bite 20 times. You may need to keep a week or two of food records (page 21).
4. **Develop a positive attitude.** Many people join a weight loss program to feel they belong to a group and to get encouragement. Celebrate your ability and every success.

Chapter 10
EATING OUT

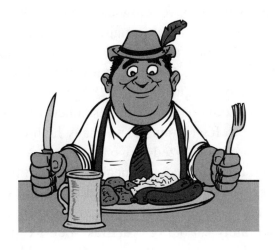

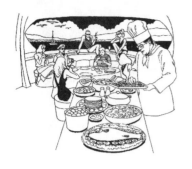

*I*s eating out in restaurants a challenge?

▼
TIP:

Yes—for everyone. Several studies show that eating out makes it almost impossible to have a low-calorie day. One study showed the group who most often ate at restaurants consumed 30% more calories per day, 5% more fat, and 36% less fiber compared to those who ate out the least often. A second study showed that those who ate in restaurants most frequently ate 228 more calories, 19 more grams of fat, more sodium, and much less fiber per day. If you go there, you will eat it. Restaurants serve many high-calorie foods, and the servings are super-sized or worse yet, all-you-can-eat buffets. Lunches are often full-course meals. The more frequently you eat out, the more you need advanced level restaurant skills (page 97). To be successful with weight management, cook at home most of the time, and rarely eat out or order take-out. Keep in mind, you don't have to cook like Martha Stewart. Many cookbooks offer quick, easy, healthy recipes.

*W*hat are the restaurant skills
I need for eating out and
keeping on my weight loss plan?

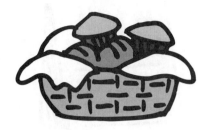

▼
TIP:

*P*lan ahead. Step 1: Choose a restaurant that offers healthy choices. If you don't know what's on the menu, call ahead, stop by for a copy, or request a faxed copy. Step 2: Set a calorie goal for the meal. Use your weekly food records to see if you can afford a calorie splurge. Step 3: Ask about food preparation and serving sizes before you order. How is the item prepared (in butter, oil, fried)? Can you request special preparation (broiled, steamed, no butter)? Are low-calorie salad dressings available? What is the soup base (water, milk, cream)? What comes with the entrée (French fries, coleslaw)? Can you request items not on the menu or substitute healthier items? Can you have a child's serving?

Actions to take:

- Carry low-calorie dressings with you.
- Put half the order in a doggie bag before you start to eat.
- Split the entrée or dessert with someone.
- Remove bread, crackers, chips, or rolls from the table.
- Carry items to round out the meal, such as fresh fruit or raw vegetables to go with a turkey sandwich.
- Walk to and from the restaurant to burn some calories.

What are some tips for placing an order in restaurants?

▼
TIP:

Look for ways to increase the amount of food and nutrition, but not the fat and calories. Try these:

- Construct a meal without an entrée, using appetizers, soup, salad, or side vegetables. For example: shrimp cocktail, broth-based vegetable soup, baked potato, steamed vegetable.
- Order without looking at the menu.
- Order items not listed on the menu, such as a steamed vegetable plate.
- Replace high-fat items with low-fat items (baked potato for French fries, tossed salad for coleslaw).
- Request sauces on the side—dip your fork into the sauce, and then into the food.
- Order double portions of salad and vegetable.
- Make special requests for low-fat preparation—no added fat to fish or vegetables.
- Order at least 2 cups of vegetables without fat with your meal. (Corn and potatoes are not counted as vegetables.)
- Order the smaller lunch size or early-bird special portion.
- When sharing a meal with your dining companion, order an extra potato or vegetable.
- Ask that only one roll or breadstick be brought with your salad.
- Become a regular customer; you'll most likely get what you request.

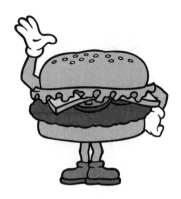

How does fast food figure into my weight management?

▼
TIP:

It may not fit. A recent study looked at three commonly ordered take-out meals from three different fast food chains. The typical meal from these fast food restaurants had more than 1,000 calories in the meal. Authors concluded that eating even one fast food meal a week made it extremely difficult for the participants to meet their recommended health guidelines. Another analysis has reported the calories of an average fast food meal at 1,300 calories. And that was before you super-sized the meal for only 80 cents more. Once super-sized, the final tally was 1,660 calories for lunch! Very few people can afford 1,600 calories for lunch on a regular basis, yet this is the world we live in. You have to be creative and find ways to cut calories. Don't get super-sizes; they cost you too much. There are some lower-calorie choices available in fast food chains, such as grilled chicken sandwiches and entrée salads with low-calorie dressings. In all fast food restaurants, try to stay away from anything that is fried or covered in cheese or sauce. If those are the only choices, go for smaller servings. Making the right choice when placing your order is the key!

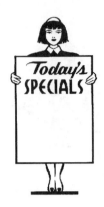

How can I work in my favorite foods when eating out?

▼
TIP:

According to successful weight managers, "if you want it, have it." You need to break away from good food/bad food thinking. The message is simple: when you have treats, enjoy them. You don't have to feel guilty. But—plan, plan, plan. "If you fail to plan, you plan to fail." Identify the food that is important to you, and figure how many calories are in the serving it will take for you to enjoy that food. Using that calorie figure, figure what else can be included in the meal, if anything. Add up the calories you need to save up for the treat. Figure what your usual calories would be at that meal, and subtract them from the calories in the treat meal. If you usually eat 450 calories at lunch, but your favorite food is 950 calories, you have 500 extra calories to fit into your week. You need to save ahead for this favorite food. Don't try to take the 500 calories from the other meals in that same day. Better to cut some calories each day for several days before the treat. Don't forget that you can burn calories with exercise, too. It all counts.

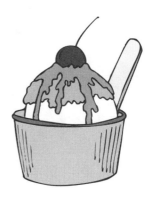

*C*an you give an example of how to save
up calories for a treat?

▼

TIP:

H ere is a woman who weighs 180 lbs. To maintain her weight,
her daily calorie level is 1,980. Her favorite food is a Hot
Fudge Sundae, which is made with 1 cup premium ice cream (600),
1/4 cup hot fudge sauce (240), and 1/4 cup whipped cream (200).
This sundae has 1,040 calories. To create "space" for this treat, this
woman is willing to eat lightly earlier in the day and to do physical
activity twice that day, or also on the days before, to make this work.

Her day might look like this.

	Subtotals
Before Breakfast: Walked 2.5 miles = burned 300 calories	−300
Breakfast: 300 calories, including fruit and low-fat yogurt	300
Lunch: 2 (300-calorie) frozen entrées	
Plus 1 cup vegetables (40 calories)	640
Mid-afternoon: Walked 3 miles = burned 360 calories	−360
Supper: 600-calorie meal, not including the sundae	880
8 oz broiled whitefish with lemon (200)	
6 oz baked potato (120)	
2 Tbsp. sour cream (60)	
1 cup steamed vegetable (no oil) (40)	
1 oz roll (80)	
1 Tbsp butter (100)	
Hot Fudge Sundae	1040
Total Calories In	2580
Calories Out (physical activity) (300 + 360)	−660
Net Calories In	1920

SECTION IV
Excess

Chapter 11
ENVIRONMENT
OUT OF CONTROL

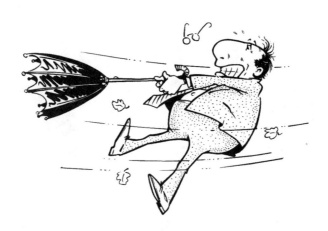

I *crave carbohydrates. Am I a carbohydrate addict?*

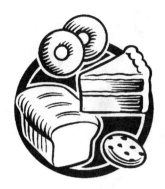

▼

TIP:

Fresh fruit, vegetables, and beans are carbohydrates, yet no one seems to be addicted to them. It is the soft, fluffy, sugar- and fat-bearing carbohydrates that cause trouble. Write down what you crave—is it doughnuts, French fries, or candy bars? Carbohydrate craving or addiction describes how eating carbohydrate triggers your appetite and a desire for more carbohydrate. If it's an addiction, you can do something about it.

Your body breaks down carbohydrate foods to glucose. The pancreas produces insulin to help body cells take in glucose and use it for energy. Some people restrict the amount of carbohydrate they eat, thinking this reduces the craving, but you need carbohydrate to feel satisfied. Some studies suggest that choosing natural or unprocessed carbohydrates, such as oatmeal or baked beans, that have more fiber helps stop cravings. Fiber makes you feel full. There's no fiber in one (or even five) doughnuts. Raw vegetables and whole fruits, such as apples, can be filling and are rich in fiber. Get some insight on your craving by keeping a diary of how your eating pattern is related to your appetite.

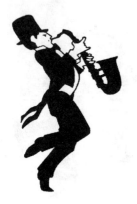

How can I lose weight when I have to eat on the run?

▼
TIP:

Plan ahead for good food choices and make use of every opportunity. It's easier to eat vegetables with ready-to-eat produce options such as pre-washed bagged salad greens and peeled baby carrots. You may save time and money by bringing a frozen low-calorie entree to pop into the workplace microwave or raw vegetables and fruit from home. You can build more physical activity into each day by taking a 5-minute break to walk around. As you go through your day, watch for opportunities to walk more. Use a pedometer and add a few extra steps each day. Many people gain weight because time for eating a balanced diet and being physically active becomes a lower priority than work or other activities. Nothing is more important than your health, exercising, and eating right. Get your priorities straight, and you can create time to take care of yourself.

To avoid confusion and indecision, set clear goals to help keep yourself organized. For example, eat an apple a day. Take the stairs. Have a salad for dinner. Make a shopping list. Cook dinner.

*H*ow can I say no to friends who push
food?

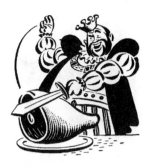

▼
TIP:

It's hard to say "No" when food is offered to you by friends and
family. People can be offended when you reject the food they
offer. Food has many emotional meanings. Mothers often express
their love for their families by cooking favorite meals. We socialize
with friends and family over foods. Say "no, thank you" firmly and
clearly. Talking to others about how they can help is the first step in
helping them understand that managing your weight is important to
you. Sometimes you can suggest other foods. You can take a small
piece. Serious food pushers may not respond to more subtle
approaches. Then you have to be more firm and resort to tactics
that are more direct. You may need to say, "I feel that I have trouble
controlling my weight and my health when I eat with you. Please
support me in my decision to avoid eating seconds (or whatever you
have decided to do)." If you can get them on your side, you'll both
win.

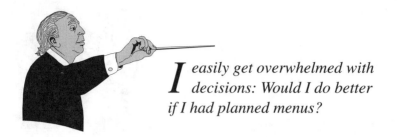

I easily get overwhelmed with decisions: Would I do better if I had planned menus?

TIP:

Yes. Studies have shown that people can achieve long-term success using menus or prepackaged foods. They help if you feel you need more structure, for example getting started, when you are under stress, and when you have slipped or gained back some weight.

Making food choices can be difficult when you are trying to break old habits. Using menus or packaged foods can make your decisions easier. ADA publishes the Month-of-Meals series of books to provide you with millions of menus. You can choose a cuisine and calorie level suited to your needs.

If you find yourself thinking "I cannot wait until I finish this diet," you have a high risk of going back to your old habits. You may find that you will always need menus to keep you on track. If you use prepackaged meal supplements (page 24), make sure you don't round out the meal with old high-calorie snacks. If you have a shake or bar for one or two meals a day, you may find that you are hungry. Try to satisfy that hunger with raw vegetables or a piece of fruit as snacks.

When my favorite foods are around, I just cannot stay away from them. How can I stay on my meal plan?

▼
TIP:

Dealing with tempting food can be overwhelming, especially if the food is highly visible. These techniques may help you:

- Give away or freeze tempting leftovers from special celebrations.
- Avoid buying or making the food that you find so overwhelming.
- If you buy tempting foods, get the smallest size. Get the small cup or cone of ice cream rather than bringing home a half gallon.
- Negotiate with household members to keep the tempting foods out of sight or to choose other foods that are less tempting to you. For example, they could choose a type of chocolate bar that you don't like.
- Try to learn to be satisfied with a smaller serving of the tempting food. Eat slowly and focus on the taste.
- Try to find some new favorite foods that are better for your waistline.
- Talk, dance, laugh, or walk somewhere away from the food.

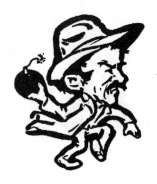

*W*hy would my husband (or my friend)
try to sabotage my diet?

▼
TIP:

If family members and friends try to lure you away or criticize your weight loss efforts, you can feel sabotaged. Let them know that you feel discouraged by their words or actions. Discuss what they can do to truly support your weight loss effort.

Think about your goals and how your weight loss may change your relationships. Sometimes the saboteur enjoys eating and wants you to be a partner in the fun of feasting. State your goals clearly to show that you are seriously trying to change the way you eat. What are their goals for you? Sometime friends and family feel a conflict. They want your success, but may feel imposed upon if you request they keep tempting foods out of the house. You may need to negotiate an acceptable plan.

If your family and friends are aware of their ambivalent feelings about your weight loss, you may be able to talk about their views of the pros and cons. But many times the person sabotaging your effort is unaware of it. If you have difficulty talking with him or her, you might discuss the problem with a professional counselor or your health care provider.

Chapter 12
EMOTIONS AND
ROADBLOCKS

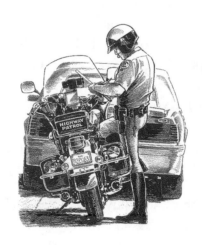

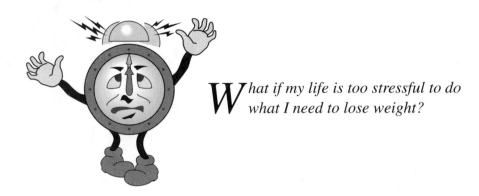

What if my life is too stressful to do what I need to lose weight?

It is important to identify the reasons for the stress and plan ways to reduce it or manage it. The things you can do to relieve stress—such as exercising and making healthy food choices (for the vitamins and minerals that help you manage stress) are the very things you need for weight loss, too. You can actually work on weight loss and lowering stress at the same time. Take 30 minutes to write down the stresses on you and some things to do to manage them. Breathe deeply. Take a yoga class. Punch a pillow. Run around the block. Walk every day. Read a book. You need balance in your life. Otherwise you'll do what many people do—eat more and exercise less, and actually gain weight. If you learn to reset your goals to hold your weight steady during high stress and then refocus on weight loss when your stress level is reduced, you may be more successful.

If you have diabetes, any physical stress (cold, flu, infection, or injury) or emotional stress can raise your blood sugar levels. Overeating and skipping exercise will just raise them higher. Start to defuse the stresses in your life today.

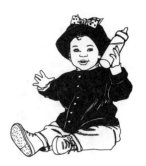

I use food to comfort and nurture myself
when I'm feeling angry, depressed, or
upset. Will this habit prevent me from being
successful with weight loss?

▼
TIP:

Not as long as you are aware of what you're doing and can find
other ways to comfort and nurture yourself. Overeating in
response to negative feelings is called emotional eating. Emotional
eaters use food to cope when they feel angry or upset, anxious,
worried, tense, depressed, disappointed, or discouraged. Other
people lose their appetite and eat less in response to these same
emotions. There are several reasons people develop the habit of
emotional eating; eating tends to calm mood. Children are often
conditioned to associate eating with being soothed or nurtured.
Eating is a quick, convenient way to temporarily distract yourself
from stressful emotions. There is nothing wrong with eating food
for emotional reasons. The problem with eating for emotional reasons is that many people do it in a chaotic manner, often overeating
in an attempt to push down or blot out feelings. This behavior pattern can make you feel numb, guilty, and out of control, which can
make it difficult to manage your weight and control your blood sugars. You may need to see a counselor for help with changing this
habit.

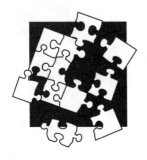

How can I change my tendency to eat in response to negative emotions, so I can make better progress with weight loss?

▼ TIP:

First, ask yourself the following questions:

1. Is emotional eating causing me problems with overeating, weight control, or blood sugar control?
2. What kind of events, situations, people, and feelings trigger this response?
3. How does emotional eating affect my physical well-being, diabetes control, self-esteem, and mood after I've eaten?
4. What else besides eating can I choose that may also calm my mood or distract me from stressful emotions?

Share your feelings with someone else or your journal rather than stuffing them down with food. Take a walk or do some other exercise that you enjoy—this also improves your mood and distracts you. If you are tired, take a nap rather than eating to stay awake. You're likely to feel better with rest. Try to address the problem causing the negative emotions and work out a plan to deal with it. If you do eat, acknowledge how you feel and give yourself permission to eat in a positive, mindful, deliberate way. You may find that a smaller portion of food helps you feel better and still allows you success with losing weight and controlling your blood sugars.

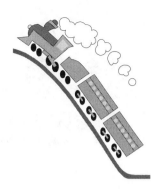

I've tried so many diets and failed. How can I face weight loss again without a sense of hopelessness?

▼
TIP:

First, work on your attitude. View your past experiences with weight loss as a wealth of information about what works for you and what doesn't. Evaluate what programs worked best for you and what in your life made you lose focus and regain weight. Make a list of things that were helpful. For example, when you exercised on the way home from work, you were more consistent, and you snacked less before dinner. Maybe a regular afternoon snack prevented you from getting too hungry and overeating at dinner.

Give yourself credit for all your "small wins." Changing your lifestyle and losing weight is not easy, and it takes a lot of time and effort. If you break your effort into smaller steps, you will set yourself up for success. For example, you set a goal to walk 30 minutes 3 times a week and decide you can do that. Give yourself credit for a small win each time you walk. If you decide to eat at least 3 servings of fruits and vegetables each day and you do it, be proud. Don't wait until you reach your goal weight to celebrate success. Each pound you lose is progress!

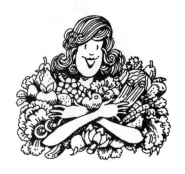

I like to eat a lot. How can I keep from feeling deprived?

If you are feeling deprived, you don't have a meal plan that can become a lifelong habit. Yours may not have enough volume of food. Other times a feeling of deprivation comes from trying to avoid favorite foods or saying "no" when others are feasting. No matter what is causing you to feel deprived, you need to develop a new way of thinking about your relationship with food and move from feeling deprived to feeling satisfied. If you need volume, focus on eating lots of low-calorie foods that are filling, such as vegetables and low-fat carbs. Salads and a broth-based soup can make you feel full and satisfied. Books that help you think about food volume as a way to feel more satisfied include *Dr. Shapiro's Picture Perfect Weight Loss: The Visual Program for Permanent Weight Loss* by Howard Shapiro and *The Volumetrics Weight Control Plan: Feel Full on Fewer Calories* by Barbara Rolls and Robert Barnett. You can plan ahead so you can eat a favorite food or meal by saving calories. Having your favorite foods is easier when you learn to appreciate small servings of them.

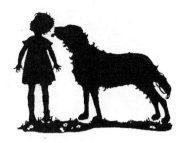

*W*hen I diet, I start feeling depressed. What can I do to keep from feeling this way?

▼
TIP:

You need to look at what may be causing the depressed feeling. If you are feeling deprived or you are losing weight quickly but feel out of sorts and irritable, you may be eating too little. Starvation studies have shown that severely restricting the amount of food eaten can cause depression. Your body may react to a very-low-calorie weight loss diet as starvation. Increasing your calorie level by 200 or 300 calories may improve your mood. Increasing physical activity improves mood, too.

If you are not losing weight, your depressed feeling may be associated with working hard to lose weight without seeing any results of your work. Be patient and speak well of yourself and your efforts. Make this a new powerful habit for dealing with depression. No matter what the cause of your depressed mood, you may find talking to a counselor helpful. Some social workers and psychologists specialize in weight control management. Your health professional may be able to recommend one for you.

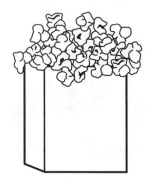

*W*hat can I do when I get the munchies?

Try a delay-and-distract strategy. Drinking a glass of water or going for a walk can keep you busy until the urge passes. Delay and distract may help with eating out of boredom. Forbidden food lists often make the food to be avoided very attractive. Eating a little serving can satisfy a craving as well as removing the temptation.

Hormones in pregnancy or PMS can trigger the munchies as can some medications or illicit drugs such as marijuana. This may occur as a craving for a specific food such as chocolate. If a medication is causing your appetite, your physician may be able to prescribe a different drug.

Food cravings are NOT your body's way of preventing nutritional deficiency. Eating a well-balanced diet and a small portion of the craved food, such as chocolate, may help control cravings that are hormonally triggered. Sometimes two foods are linked and eating one triggers a craving for the other. You can choose other foods or learn to eat one without the other. For example, if you always eat bread with butter, you can avoid both, choose a different kind of bread to enjoy without butter, or eat only a small portion.

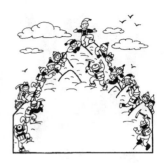

*W*hat can I do to keep motivated
about eating healthfully?

▼
TIP:

*H*ere are some ideas to help you:

1. **Build your confidence that you can succeed.** You have to
   believe in yourself to succeed at anything you do. Talking or
   thinking of yourself negatively is a common pitfall. Learn from
   slips. Practice making positive self-statements to yourself and
   out loud.
2. **Build in rewards.** You need to be good to yourself. Food is not
   the only reward. It is easy to use high-calorie "comfort" foods to
   help deal with stress. Look for non-food rewards such as a new
   CD or a visit to a museum or park. Also, buy fresh produce,
   which tastes so good that it's really a treat.
3. **Think in small steps.** Set small goals that you can measure.
   Feel good about your accomplishments, such as going for a walk
   even though you were tired. Don't get discouraged by the scale.
   Losing 1/2 to 1 pound a week is a healthy rate of weight loss.
4. **Avoid getting too hungry.** A common pitfall is trying to go all
   day without food. It may be easy to skip meals during the day
   when you are busy, but you are at risk for a nightly food binge.
   Treat yourself to breakfast and lunch.

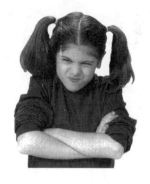

Why does everybody keep nagging me when I am trying to diet? Don't they know that it makes me not even want to try to lose weight?

▼
TIP:

Friends, family, and co-workers can be annoying when they provide unwanted guidance or advice. Comments such as, "You can't have that . . ." can make you feel like a child who has to get permission to eat. Even gentle reminders about your plan can make you feel resentful. You can take charge by letting people know how to change their negative support into positive support. Make a list of what you want people to do or say to help boost your motivation. For example, having a walking partner may be helpful. You may want praise for making good choices. On the other hand, you may feel you are being treated like a child. Keeping snack food out of sight may be helpful or it could make you feel left out. Some people want everybody to ignore their weight loss efforts. Only you can decide whether comments and actions are helpful or harmful. After you decide, share with friends, family, and co-workers what you want them to do to support you.

Chapter 13
INSURANCE
AND ADVOCACY

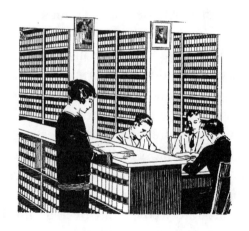

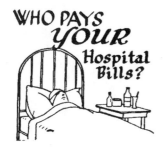

WHO PAYS *your* Hospital Bills?

D *oes insurance reimburse for obesity treatment?*

▼

TIP:

While reimbursement for diabetes self-management training and medical nutrition therapy in general is improving, treatment for obesity is usually not covered by third party payers. If you have other health conditions that accompany the obesity (page 9), the chances for being reimbursed for treatment are improved. Some companies make decisions based on individual patient situations. Others have a set policy regardless of who the patient is and what their medical conditions are. Ask your insurance carriers about what coverage is available. Mention all your medical diagnoses other than obesity. For example, "my doctor has recommended I participate in this comprehensive lifestyle change program for the treatment of my diabetes, high blood pressure, and high cholesterol." Portions of obesity treatment that are most likely eligible for coverage are physician visits and lab work. Insurance companies do not reimburse for nutritional supplements used for obesity treatment, and prescriptions are rarely covered. Coverage for the maintenance phase of a weight management program is usually not covered.

As of January 2002, Medical Nutrition Therapy (MNT) to control diabetes is covered for patients with diabetes.

*H*ow can I become an advocate for a better environment to reduce obesity?

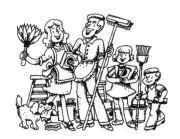

▼
TIP:

We have an abundance of food, which is aggressively marketed in mass media. Extra-large portions of food promote high-calorie consumption. But no one gets extra portions of physical activity. We need to:

- Reduce television, videotape, and video game use by children.
- Lobby local schools for more fruits and vegetables and fewer high-fat foods in the cafeteria.
- Restore daily physical education classes and team sports opportunities in schools.

Changes in the community to promote physical activity may offer the most practical approach to prevent obesity. Simple changes such as improving the appearance of stairwells and adding sidewalks and bicycle trails in work, school, shopping, and residential areas will really help. Replacing automobile trips with walking or bicycling is the best way to increase physical activity in communities.

To make our communities healthier places to live we need a partnership that includes food marketers and manufacturers, public and private purchasers of health care, large employers, transportation agencies, urban planners, and real-estate developers.

Chapter 14
RESOURCES

Y ou can get help from several reputable web sites that focus on weight loss. Some good choices include:

www.cyberdiet.com This site was developed by registered dietitians and features a personalized menu planner, recipes, exercise information, and other useful information to assist in weight loss. They charge a fee.

www.weightwatchers.com or *www.123athome.com* The Weight Watchers web site features their commercial weight loss programs, meeting locations, a message board, recipe swap, and a weight loss readiness assessment.

www.TOPS.org Take Off Pounds Sensibly (TOPS) is a not-for-profit organization and its web site features a list of local chapters, weight loss tips, and communications via message board and chat room.

www.learneducation.com The Lifestyle, Exercise, Attitudes, Relationships, and Nutrition (LEARN) web site features the educational materials developed by Dr. Kelly Brownell, self-assessments for binge eating, weight loss readiness, and stress management readiness.

www.kidsfood.org The Kid CyberCafe web site was developed by the Connecticut Association of Human Services to provides a variety of activities for kids, parents, and teachers with emphasis on 3rd through 5th grades.

www.familyfoodzone.com The Family Food Zone web site is sponsored by the National Dairy Council. Features include the idea of the day, quick meal ideas, an interactive food pyramid, teacher information, and kid cooking.

Other web sites that provide useful information include the American Diabetes Association at *www.diabetes.org* and The American Dietetic Association at *www.eatright.org*.

RDs can provide medical nutrition therapy, to address nutrition issues in the overall treatment of a medical condition. While weight loss counseling is often not included in insurance plans, a growing number of insurance companies provide coverage for diabetes medical nutrition therapy. You may want to find an RD who is also a certified diabetes educator (CDE) using national web sites that include local information. The American Dietetic Association's web site *www.eatright.org* provides a listing of RDs and the American Association of Diabetes Educators web site *www.aadenet.org* lists RDs and other members.

INDEX

▼

U.S. Department of Agriculture (USDA), 14, 92

Vacations, 82
Variety, 88, 94
Vegetables, 14, 17–18, 22, 24, 26, 45, 90, 92, 105, 108
Very low calorie diets (VLCDs), 23, 32, 117
Vitamins, 89–90

Waist-to-hip measurement, 9, 10, 43, 47
Walking, 69, 77, 106, 112, 120

Warm up, 50, 71
Water, 53, 93, 118
Weighing, 41
Weight, 3–12
Weight management program, 19–20
Weight loss, 3, 27, 31, 34–35, 37
Weight loss drugs, 62
Western lifestyle, 12, 37
Whole grains, 17
Willpower, 87

About the American Diabetes Association

The American Diabetes Association is the nation's leading voluntary health organization supporting diabetes research, information, and advocacy. Its mission is to prevent and cure diabetes and to improve the lives of all people affected by diabetes. The American Diabetes Association is the leading publisher of comprehensive diabetes information. Its huge library of practical and authoritative books for people with diabetes covers every aspect of self-care—cooking and nutrition, fitness, weight control, medications, complications, emotional issues, and general self-care.

To order American Diabetes Association books: Call 1-800-232-6733. Or log on to http://store.diabetes.org

To join the American Diabetes Association: Call 1-800-806-7801. www.diabetes.org/membership

For more information about diabetes or ADA programs and services: Call 1-800-342-2383. E-mail: Customerservice@diabetes.org or log on to www.diabetes.org

To locate an ADA/NCQA Recognized Provider of quality diabetes care in your area: Call 1-703-549-1500 ext. 2202. www.diabetes.org/recognition/Physicians/List All.asp

To find an ADA Recognized Education Program in your area: Call 1-888-232-0822. www.diabetes.org/recognition/education.asp

To join the fight to increase funding for diabetes research, end discrimination, and improve insurance coverage: Call 1-800-342-2383. www.diabetes.org/advocacy

To find out how you can get involved with the programs in your community: Call 1-800-342-2383. See below for program Web addresses.

- *American Diabetes Month:* Educational activities aimed at those diagnosed with diabetes—month of November. www.diabetes.org/ADM
- *American Diabetes Alert:* Annual public awareness campaign to find the undiagnosed—held the fourth Tuesday in March. www.diabetes.org/alert
- *The Diabetes Assistance & Resources Program (DAR):* diabetes awareness program targeted to the Latino community. www.diabetes.org/DAR
- *African American Program:* diabetes awareness program targeted to the African American community. www.diabetes.org/africanamerican
- *Awakening the Spirit: Pathways to Diabetes Prevention & Control:* diabetes awareness program targeted to the Native American community. www.diabetes.org/awakening

To find out about an important research project regarding type 2 diabetes: www.diabetes.org/ada/research.asp

To obtain information on making a planned gift or charitable bequest: Call 1-888-700-7029. www.diabetes.org/ada/plan.asp

To make a donation or memorial contribution: Call 1-800-342-2383. www.diabetes.org/ada/cont.asp